Infections and Male Infertility: General Pathophysiology Diagnosis, and Treatment

(Part I)

Authored by

Sulagna Dutta
Basic Medical Sciences Department
College of Medicine
Ajman University, Ajman
UAE

&

Pallav Sengupta
Department of Biomedical Sciences
College of Medicine
Gulf Medical University, Ajman
UAE

Infections and Male Infertility: General Pathophysiology, Diagnosis, and Treatment

(Part 1)

Authors: Sulagna Dutta and Pallav Sengupta

ISBN (Online): 978-981-5305-30-2

ISBN (Print): 978-981-5305-31-9

ISBN (Paperback): 978-981-5305-32-6

©2025, Bentham Books imprint.

Published by Bentham Science Publishers Pte. Ltd. Singapore. All Rights Reserved.

First published in 2025.

need for a court order if at any point you breach any terms of this License Agreement. In no event will any delay or failure by Bentham Science Publishers in enforcing your compliance with this License Agreement constitute a waiver of any of its rights.

3. You acknowledge that you have read this License Agreement, and agree to be bound by its terms and conditions. To the extent that any other terms and conditions presented on any website of Bentham Science Publishers conflict with, or are inconsistent with, the terms and conditions set out in this License Agreement, you acknowledge that the terms and conditions set out in this License Agreement shall prevail.

Bentham Science Publishers Pte. Ltd.
80 Robinson Road #02-00
Singapore 068898
Singapore
Email: subscriptions@benthamscience.net

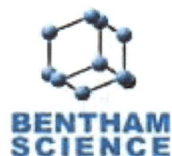

BENTHAM SCIENCE

CONTENTS

FOREWORD

The realm of medical science is both vast and perpetually developing, embodying a myriad of interconnected specialties, each illuminating distinct aspects of truth while also preserving their own unresolved mysteries. Various subfields of male infertility, previously obscured by bias and misconceptions, have now emerged as topics of high research interest. The importance of understanding the underlying mechanisms of male infertility is being increasingly acknowledged, yet certain gaps in knowledge persist, particularly in understanding the intricate role that infections play in male infertility. *'Infections and Male Infertility: Part I: General Pathophysiology, Diagnosis, and Treatment'*, penned by Dr. Sulagna Dutta and Dr. Pallav Sengupta, serves as an enlightening exploration into this multifaceted domain.

This pivotal composition amalgamates sound scientific research with clinical insight to unravel the complex association between infections and male infertility. By employing this method, Drs. Dutta and Sengupta shed light on the influence of infections on the pathophysiology of male infertility, a subject that is often neglected but critical to a comprehensive grasp of the field. It possesses the potential to reshape our viewpoints and, possibly, our medical practices.

The authors' extensive expertise and experience resonate throughout the text, emphasizing the significance of their contributions. Their committed review of the current literature and original research helps bridge a crucial gap in the field. The organization of the book—initiating with an exhaustive investigation into the general pathophysiology of male infertility, transitioning into the role of infections, and concluding with the diagnosis and treatment of these conditions—provides a graduated learning journey that is both intellectually invigorating and pragmatically applicable.

The true value of this work goes beyond mere academic rigor. By focusing on infection-induced male infertility, an area often fraught with misunderstanding and insufficient research, Drs. Dutta and Sengupta present comprehensive views on male fertility. Through an exhaustive discussion, they delve into various aspects of infection conditions, inflammatory processes, and the complex interactions between infection, inflammation, endocrine systems, and reproduction. Their insights not only enable more nuanced conversations and interventions but also pave the way for the scientific community, researchers, students, and general readers who are more informed on these critical subjects.

'Infections and Male Infertility: Part I: General Pathophysiology, Diagnosis and Treatment' functions not only as a rich repository of scientific data but also as a reflection of the progressive evolution of our shared understanding of reproductive health. It embodies the scientific and societal obligation to dissect intricate interactions and to perpetually seek a more refined comprehension of human reproductive immunology.

Whether you are an established medical professional, a researcher, a novice embarking on your academic journey in reproductive medicine, or an inquisitive reader, this publication promises to inform, question, and inspire.

As we immerse ourselves in this text, let us recollect the statement by William Osler, *'Medicine is a science of uncertainty and an art of probability.'* Here's to the anticipation of scientific discoveries and the skillful practice of medicine, as steered by the trailblazing work of Dr. Sulagna Dutta and Dr. Pallav Sengupta.

Shubhadeep Roychoudhury
Department of Life Science and Bioinformatics
Assam University Silchar, India

PREFACE

The intricate subject of male infertility has, for an extended period, engaged the attention of the medical community in a mix of intrigue and difficulty. With immense excitement, we present our work titled '*Infections and Male Infertility: Part I: General Pathophysiology, Diagnosis, and Treatment*', which is a thorough investigation into one of the frequently underappreciated origins of male infertility.

The intent of this book is to provide an all-encompassing examination of the complex correlation between infectious diseases and male infertility. Our goal is to deliver a lucid narrative that transitions from the molecular interactions at the level of pathophysiology to the broader clinical outcomes of these interactions.

Drawing upon a broad spectrum of scientific inquiry, our book delves into the underlying mechanisms through which a variety of infections may perturb the male reproductive system. The biochemical pathways, immunological reactions, and genetic modifications that participate in this process are meticulously elaborated upon to elucidate this complex issue. The book endeavors to establish a theoretical and practical link between the origins of infections and their clinical implications for male fertility.

We hold the conviction that a precise diagnosis is the cornerstone of effective therapeutic intervention. In line with this, our text outlines numerous diagnostic methodologies, their deployment, and interpretation within the context of infections inducing male infertility. By clarifying these techniques, we aim to empower clinicians to better recognize and comprehend the etiology of male infertility.

The concluding segment centers on the most recent therapeutic strategies. We illuminate the contemporary cutting-edge treatments, their advantages, and restrictions while accentuating potential directions for forthcoming interventions. The book particularly emphasizes the need for a tailored, patient-centric approach to managing this condition.

This publication serves a two-fold purpose: It offers an advanced reference for medical professionals, equipping them with a deeper insight into the sophisticated interaction between infections and male infertility. Concurrently, it offers a roadmap for researchers, laying the groundwork for future investigations into the pathophysiology, diagnosis, and treatment of infections leading to male infertility.

The process of creating this book proved to be both demanding and fulfilling. We express our gratitude to the many researchers and clinicians whose invaluable contributions have set the stage for this exhaustive analysis. With the publication of this work, we aspire to ignite further research and discussion, thereby paving the way to enhanced diagnostic and therapeutic strategies for male infertility.

We appreciate your companionship in this exploration of a relatively uncharted facet of reproductive medicine. We trust that '*Infections and Male Infertility: Part I: General Pathophysiology, Diagnosis, and Treatment*' will amplify your comprehension of this intricate domain and encourage ongoing research, innovation, and improvement in patient care.

Sulagna Dutta
Basic Medical Sciences Department
College of Medicine
Ajman University
Ajman, UAE

&

Pallav Sengupta
Department of Biomedical Sciences
College of Medicine
Gulf Medical University
Ajman, UAE

CHAPTER 1

Male Infertility and its Causes

Abstract: Male infertility, defined as the inability to achieve conception after a year of unprotected intercourse, is an imperative global issue. Understanding its etiology is vital for effective diagnosis, treatment, and support. The chapter provides a comprehensive overview of the anatomy and physiology of the male reproductive system, addressing the causes of male infertility. It begins by introducing male infertility and stressing the importance of investigating its causes. An extensive examination of the male reproductive system follows, encompassing structural attributes, functionalities, and endocrine regulation. The chapter identifies genetic factors, environmental exposures, lifestyle choices, and pathological conditions as critical contributors to male infertility. Additionally, it explores the psychological toll of infertility, highlighting emotional distress and coping strategies while emphasizing the importance of professional and social support. The chapter concludes by discussing innovative research and treatment avenues, including genomics, epigenomics, proteomics, metabolomics, and spermatogonial stem cell therapy as promising fields. The roles of assisted reproductive technologies, male contraception, and lifestyle and environmental factors are also evaluated. This chapter underscores male infertility as a complex issue with a heterogeneous etiology and aims to foster an in-depth understanding and improve reproductive health outcomes for affected individuals and couples.

Keywords: Diet, Epididymis, Erectile Dysfunction, Exercise, Hypothalamus, Infections, Inhibins, Male Infertility, Prostate Gland, Radiation, Retrograde Ejaculation, Smoking, Spermatogenesis, Spermiogenesis, Sperm Capacitation, Steroidogenesis, Temperature, Testis, Testosterone, Toxins, Varicocele.

INTRODUCTION

Infertility, a term that bears emotional connotations for many, is a common medical issue affecting approximately 15% of couples worldwide. Among these, nearly half can be attributed to male infertility [1]. Male infertility, in the simplest terms, is defined as the inability of a man to cause pregnancy in a fertile female after a year of unprotected intercourse [2]. It has myriad causes that span from physical and psychological to genetic and environmental. As our understanding of these factors continues to deepen, we hope to improve not only the diagnosis but also the treatment options available to affected individuals.

The importance and prevalence of male infertility are often underestimated in societal discussions around fertility, which typically focus more on women. However, this issue holds substantial weight as it affects a significant proportion of men globally. The World Health Organization estimates that up to 7% of men worldwide are affected by some form of infertility [3]. This percentage, though seemingly small, translates into millions of individuals and couples grappling with the often-devastating news of fertility issues. Furthermore, the male factor contributes to around 50% of all cases of infertility in couples, emphasizing the gender parity in this issue [4].

The rationale for the present chapter is multifaceted. Firstly, it aims to offer a comprehensive overview of male infertility and its causes to facilitate a broader understanding of the topic. As this is a problem with numerous contributing factors, an in-depth exploration of each cause is essential to fully grasp the complexity of male infertility. Secondly, it underscores the significance and prevalence of male infertility, attempting to recalibrate the often female-focused narrative around infertility. Finally, it hopes to provide a foundation of knowledge from which further research and treatment options can be developed, potentially benefiting millions of individuals worldwide.

In the forthcoming sections, we will delve into the biological mechanics of male infertility, outline the most common causes, and discuss the latest research findings in the field. The chapter will also shed light on the physiological, genetic, and environmental contributors to male infertility and review the existing diagnostic techniques and therapeutic interventions. By enhancing our understanding of this critical issue, we hope to contribute to the ongoing efforts to develop better strategies for diagnosis, management, and treatment of male infertility.

Definition of Male Infertility

Male infertility is defined as the inability of a man to impregnate a fertile female partner despite regular, unprotected sexual intercourse for a year or longer [5]. This can occur due to several factors, including low sperm count, poor sperm motility, abnormal sperm morphology, or a blockage in the reproductive tract. Other possible causes of male infertility include hormonal imbalances, genetic abnormalities, and certain medical conditions such as diabetes or a history of chemotherapy [6].

Importance of Understanding Male Infertility and its Causes

Understanding male infertility is essential for several reasons. First, male infertility is a widespread issue that can significantly impact the ability of a couple to conceive. Approximately 30% of infertility cases are due to male factors alone, and another 20-30% are caused by both male and female factors [4]. This highlights the need for increased awareness and understanding of male infertility, as it plays a significant role in infertility cases. Second, understanding male infertility can help identify potential causes and treatments. For example, low sperm count can be caused by a variety of factors, including lifestyle choices such as smoking, excessive alcohol consumption, and a sedentary lifestyle [7]. Identifying and addressing these factors can potentially improve the fertility of a man. Additionally, certain medical conditions or genetic abnormalities may require more advanced treatment options, such as assisted reproductive technologies (ART) [8]. Third, understanding male infertility can help alleviate the stigma surrounding infertility. Infertility can be a sensitive topic, and many men may feel ashamed or embarrassed to seek help. However, understanding that male infertility is a medical condition that affects many men can help reduce this stigma and encourage men to seek the necessary medical care.

ANATOMY AND PHYSIOLOGY OF MALE REPRODUCTIVE SYSTEM

Overview of Male Reproductive Anatomy

The male reproductive system is made up of several organs, which are responsible for producing and transporting sperm. The primary organs of the male reproductive system include the testes, epididymis, vas deferens, seminal vesicles, prostate gland, and urethra Fig. (**1**).

Testes

The testes are the primary male reproductive organs. They are responsible for producing sperm and the hormone testosterone. The testes are located in the scrotum, which is a pouch of skin that hangs below the penis. The testes are composed of numerous small, coiled tubules called seminiferous tubules, which produce sperm [9]. The Leydig cells of the testes produce testosterone [10].

Epididymis

The epididymis is a long, coiled tube located behind each testicle. It is responsible for storing sperm that have been produced in the testes until they are ready to be ejaculated. During this time, the sperm mature and gain the ability to swim [11].

Vas Deferens

The vas deferens is a muscular tube that transports mature sperm from the epididymis to the urethra. It travels from the epididymis through the inguinal canal and into the abdomen, where it passes over the bladder and joins the seminal vesicles to form the ejaculatory duct [9, 12].

Seminal Vesicles

The seminal vesicles are a pair of glands located at the base of the bladder. They secrete a fluid that makes up the majority of the volume of semen. The fluid contains fructose, which provides energy for the sperm, and other nutrients [13].

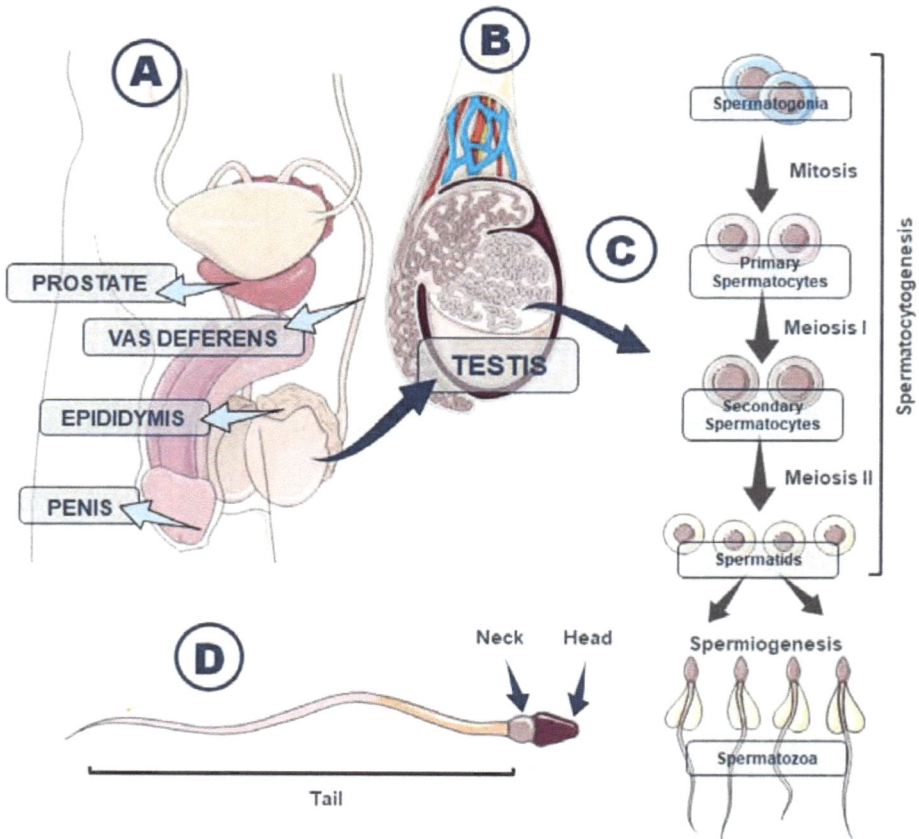

Fig. (1). Anatomy of the male reproductive system (A) indicating the organs included. (B) The primary function of the testis is to produce spermatozoa by the process of spermatogenesis, followed by sperm cell maturation in the epididymis, resulting in the development of mature spermatozoa (C).

Prostate Gland

The prostate gland is a walnut-sized gland located beneath the bladder. It surrounds the urethra, which is the tube that carries urine and semen out of the body [9]. The prostate gland secretes a fluid that helps to nourish and protect the sperm. It also helps to make the semen more alkaline, which protects the sperm from the acidic environment of the vagina [14].

Urethra

The urethra is the tube that carries urine and semen out of the body. It passes through the prostate gland and the penis. During ejaculation, the urethra carries the semen out of the male reproductive tract [15].

FUNCTIONS OF THE MALE REPRODUCTIVE SYSTEM

The male reproductive system is a complex assembly of organs and structures, including the testes, epididymis, vas deferens, seminal vesicles, prostate gland, and penis. Its primary function is the production and delivery of sperm, the male reproductive cell, into the female reproductive tract for fertilization [16].

Spermatogenesis

Spermatogenesis is the process of sperm cell production that occurs in the seminiferous tubules of the testes. It begins during puberty and continues throughout the life of a man. The process consists of three main phases: mitosis, meiosis, and spermiogenesis. In the mitotic phase, spermatogonial stem cells (SSCs), which are located in the basal compartment of the seminiferous tubules, undergo mitosis to produce two types of daughter cells: more SSCs (to maintain the stem cell pool) and primary spermatocytes [17]. This phase ensures a continuous supply of cells for spermatogenesis. During the meiotic phase, primary spermatocytes undergo meiosis I and II to form secondary spermatocytes and, subsequently, spermatids. Meiosis I, a reductional division, reduces the chromosome number from 46 (diploid) to 23 (haploid). Meiosis II, an equational division, does not alter the chromosome number but separates the sister chromatids. The end products of these two rounds of divisions are haploid spermatids [17].

Spermiogenesis

Spermiogenesis is the transformation of haploid spermatids into mature spermatozoa. It involves several morphological changes that include the formation of the acrosome (a specialized structure that contains enzymes crucial for fertilization), elongation and compaction of the nucleus, formation of the flagellum (tail), and removal of unnecessary cytoplasm. The end result is a motile sperm cell specialized for the delivery of the male genome to the egg [17, 18].

Sperm Maturation

Sperm maturation or capacitation refers to a complex biochemical process that enables sperm cells to become competent to fertilize an egg. This process involves a series of physiological changes that occur in the sperm cells as they move through the male reproductive tract, including the epididymis, vas deferens, and seminal vesicles [11, 13]. Sperm maturation or capacitation is a process that prepares sperm cells for fertilization [19]. This process involves several steps, including changes in the sperm cell membrane, the cytoskeleton, and the acrosome. The process of sperm maturation can be divided into two stages: the first stage is known as the 'pre-capacitation' stage, and the second stage is known as the 'capacitation' stage [19].

The Pre-capacitation Stage

The pre-capacitation stage is the first step in the process of sperm maturation. During this stage, the sperm cells undergo several changes that make them competent to move through the female reproductive tract. One of the significant changes that occur during this stage is the loss of cholesterol from the sperm cell membrane [20]. This loss of cholesterol leads to an increase in the fluidity of the membrane, which is essential for the sperm cells to move through the female reproductive tract. Another significant change that occurs during this stage is the reorganization of the cytoskeleton. The cytoskeleton is a network of protein fibers that gives the cell its shape and structure. During the pre-capacitation stage, the cytoskeleton undergoes a reorganization that enables the sperm cells to move more efficiently [21]. This reorganization also results in the development of the flagellum, which is the tail-like structure that enables the sperm cells to move [21, 22].

The Capacitation Stage

The second stage of sperm maturation is known as the capacitation stage. During this stage, the sperm cells undergo several changes that make them competent to fertilize an egg. One of the significant changes that occur during this stage is the activation of the cAMP-dependent protein kinase A (PKA) pathway [23]. This pathway is responsible for the phosphorylation of proteins that are involved in sperm motility, capacitation, and acrosome reaction. Another significant change that occurs during this stage is the activation of the protein tyrosine kinase (PTK) pathway. This pathway is responsible for the phosphorylation of proteins that are involved in sperm-egg binding, acrosome reaction, and zona pellucida penetration [24]. The activation of the PTK pathway also results in the release of the hyaluronidase enzyme, which is involved in breaking down the hyaluronic acid in the cumulus oophorus that surrounds the egg [23, 24].

The Importance of Sperm Maturation or Capacitation

Sperm maturation or capacitation is a crucial process for male fertility. It is essential for the sperm cells to become competent to fertilize an egg [19, 22]. Without this process, the sperm cells would not be able to move through the female reproductive tract, bind to the egg, and fertilize it. Several factors can affect the process of sperm maturation or capacitation, including environmental factors, hormonal imbalances, and genetic abnormalities [22]. These factors can lead to a decrease in male fertility and can cause infertility.

Sperm Transport and Storage

After formation, spermatozoa are transported from the seminiferous tubules to the epididymis, a convoluted tube that provides a suitable environment for sperm maturation and storage. During their transit through the epididymis, sperm acquire their motility and the ability to fertilize an egg [11]. Sperm can be stored in the epididymis for several weeks. Upon sexual arousal, mature sperm are transported from the epididymis through the vas deferens, which carries sperm to the ejaculatory duct. During ejaculation, sperm is mixed with seminal fluid from the seminal vesicles, prostate gland, and bulbourethral glands to form semen. The semen is then propelled through the urethra and out of the penis [21].

Steroidogenesis

Testosterone, the primary male sex hormone, is synthesized in the Leydig cells of the testes through a process known as steroidogenesis [25]. The process begins with the conversion of cholesterol to pregnenolone*via*the enzymatic action of P450scc. Pregnenolone is then converted to progesterone, which is subsequently transformed into androstenedione through several enzymatic steps. Androstenedione is finally converted to testosterone by the enzyme 17β-hydroxysteroid dehydrogenase. Testosterone plays a crucial role in the male reproductive system, which is described in detail in the forthcoming sections [26].

Each of these stages involves finely tuned, complex biological mechanisms regulated by a wide array of hormones and cellular signals, ensuring the continuous production, maturation, and delivery of healthy sperm cells, thereby maintaining male fertility [21]. The role of testosterone, produced by the process of steroidogenesis, underscores its importance in both initiating and maintaining these processes [10]. From the initiation of spermatogenesis in the seminiferous tubules to the storage and transport of mature sperm in the epididymis and vas deferens, every aspect of this journey is crucial for successful fertilization [17]. The production of seminal fluid by the seminal vesicles, prostate gland, and bulbourethral glands further supports the function of the mature sperm, aiding their survival and successful journey to the egg [9]. With each stage taking place in different parts of the male reproductive system, this system showcases an intricate and dynamic interaction of structure and function, underlying the propagation of life. Each step is a critical piece in the complex puzzle of human reproduction, providing profound insights into the marvels of biological design and function.

Thus, the male reproductive system is a marvel of biological engineering that performs its functions with extraordinary precision. It is an intricate network of processes that ensure the perpetuation of genetic material, thereby playing a pivotal role in the preservation of human life. From spermatogenesis and spermiogenesis to sperm transport, storage, and steroidogenesis, every function has a crucial role to play, highlighting the remarkable complexity and precision of the male reproductive system.

Hormonal Regulation of the Male Reproductive System

Hormones are the key regulators of the male reproductive system, as they govern the development and function of the testes, the accessory glands, and the external genitalia. The endocrine system, which consists of various glands that secrete hormones, controls the hormonal regulation of the male reproductive system. The hypothalamus, pituitary gland, and testes are the major components involved in this process Fig. (2).

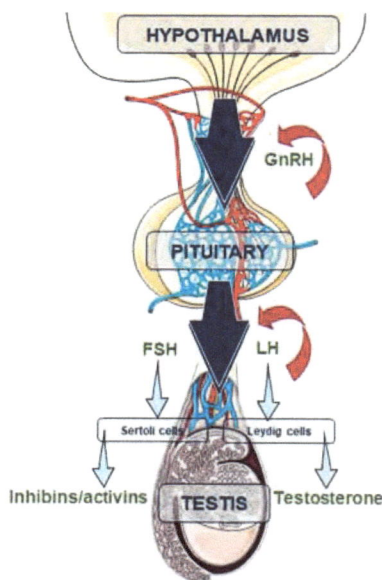

Fig. (2). Hormonal regulations of male reproductive functions.

Testicular Hormones

As discussed earlier, the testes are the primary male reproductive organs, and they are responsible for the production of testosterone, the primary male sex hormone [9]. Testosterone is secreted by the Leydig cells of the testes, and its secretion is regulated by LH secreted by the pituitary gland. LH stimulates the Leydig cells to produce testosterone, which then acts on the seminiferous tubules to regulate spermatogenesis, the process of sperm production [16]. Testosterone regulates spermatogenesis, maintains the male secondary sexual characteristics, and influences male sexual behavior. It also exerts negative feedback on the hypothalamus and pituitary gland (explained in the forthcoming sections) to regulate the secretion of gonadotropin-releasing hormone (GnRH), follicle-stimulating hormone (FSH), and luteinizing hormone (LH), thereby maintaining a balanced hormonal environment necessary for reproductive function [10]. Testosterone has several important functions in the male body. It is responsible for the development of male sexual characteristics, such as the growth of facial hair, the deepening of the voice, and the development of the penis and testes during puberty. Testosterone is also involved in the regulation of muscle mass, bone density, and the production of red blood cells [10]. In addition to testosterone, the testes also produce small amounts of other androgens, such as dehydroepiandrosterone (DHEA) and androstenedione. These androgens are converted to testosterone in peripheral tissues, and they also play a role in male sexual development and function [27].

Hypothalamic-Pituitary-Gonadal (HPG) Axis

The hypothalamus and pituitary glands are two important components of the endocrine system, which play a critical role in the regulation of the male reproductive system [16]. The hypothalamus secretes GnRH, which stimulates the pituitary gland to secrete follicle-stimulating hormones FSH and LH. These hormones then stimulate the testes to produce testosterone and regulate spermatogenesis [27].

The HPG axis is a complex feedback system, which means that the levels of hormones are constantly monitored and adjusted to maintain homeostasis. When testosterone levels are low, the hypothalamus and pituitary gland increase the production of GnRH, FSH, and LH to stimulate the testes to produce more testosterone. Conversely, when testosterone levels are high, the production of GnRH, FSH, and LH is reduced to prevent overproduction of testosterone [16]. The HPG axis is also responsible for the regulation of the male reproductive system during different stages of life. During puberty, the axis is activated to stimulate the development of male sexual characteristics, including the growth of facial and body hair, the deepening of the voice, and the development of the penis and testes. In adulthood, the HPG axis regulates the production of testosterone and sperm, as well as the maintenance of sexual function [16, 27].

Accessory Glands

The male reproductive system also includes several accessory glands, which produce secretions that contribute to the seminal fluid. These glands include the seminal vesicles, prostate gland, and bulbourethral glands [9]. The secretions from these glands provide nutrients and lubrication for the sperm, as well as a buffering capacity to protect the sperm from the acidic environment of the female reproductive tract. The secretion of these accessory gland secretions is also regulated by hormones. Testosterone and dihydrotestosterone (DHT) stimulate the secretion of the seminal vesicles and prostate gland, while estrogen stimulates the secretion of the bulbourethral glands [10]. The regulation of these secretions is important for the proper function of the male reproductive system.

CAUSES OF MALE INFERTILITY

Infertility is a condition that affects a considerable number of people worldwide. According to the World Health Organization (WHO), infertility is defined as the inability to conceive after one year of unprotected sexual intercourse [3]. Although infertility is often thought of as a female issue, male infertility is responsible for up to 50% of infertility cases [4]. The causes of male infertility are multifactorial, with a range of genetic, environmental, lifestyle, and medical factors playing a role [6] Fig. (3).

Genetic Factors

Genetic factors are an important cause of male infertility, with various genetic mutations leading to a range of reproductive abnormalities [28]. The Y chromosome is particularly relevant in male infertility, as it contains many genes involved in male reproductive development [29]. Y chromosome microdeletions, which affect a small portion of the Y chromosome, have been linked to azoospermia (absence of sperm in the ejaculate) and severe oligozoospermia (low sperm count) [30]. In addition, mutations in the cystic fibrosis transmembrane conductance regulator (CFTR) gene, which is responsible for regulating ion transport in various tissues, including the male reproductive system, can result in congenital bilateral absence of the vas deferens (CBAVD) [31]. CBAVD is a cause of obstructive azoospermia, where sperm production is normal but cannot be ejaculated due to a blockage in the vas deferens.

Other genetic abnormalities have also been linked to male infertility. For example, mutations in the androgen receptor gene can cause androgen insensitivity syndrome (AIS), where the body is unable to respond to androgen hormones. This can lead to a range of reproductive abnormalities, including hypogonadism, gynecomastia, and azoospermia [32]. Klinefelter syndrome, a condition where males have an extra X chromosome, is also associated with male infertility, with up to 80% of men with Klinefelter syndrome having azoospermia or severe oligozoospermia [33].

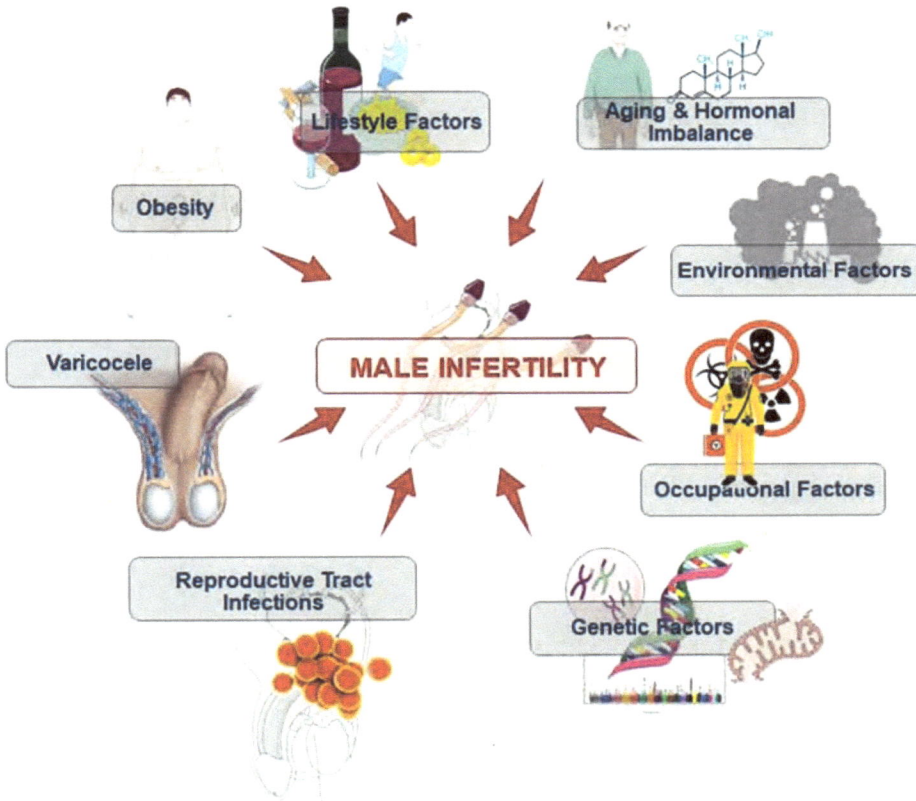

Fig. (3). Causes of male reproductive dysfunctions and infertility.

Environmental Factors

Environmental factors refer to external influences that can contribute to male infertility [34]. These factors may be chemical or physical agents that can have detrimental effects on male reproductive function. Some of the most common environmental factors that have been linked to male infertility include exposure to toxins, radiation, and extreme temperatures [6].

Toxins

Toxins are chemical substances that can have harmful effects on the male reproductive system. Exposure to environmental toxins has been linked to male infertility by causing damage to the male reproductive organs and reducing sperm count and motility [34]. Chemicals such as pesticides, heavy metals, solvents, and plastics have been implicated in male infertility [35]. For example, exposure to pesticides has been linked to reduced sperm count and motility. Similarly, heavy metals such as lead and mercury can cause DNA damage, which can lead to infertility. Plasticizers such as phthalates and bisphenol A (BPA) have also been linked to male infertility by reducing sperm count and motility [35, 36].

Radiation

Exposure to radiation can cause damage to the male reproductive organs and reduce sperm count and motility. Radiation therapy used to treat cancer can have a detrimental effect on male fertility by damaging the testes. Exposure to ionizing radiation, such as that from X-rays or nuclear accidents, can also cause DNA damage to sperm and affect male fertility [37].

Extreme Temperatures

Exposure to extreme temperatures can also affect male fertility. Prolonged exposure to high temperatures, such as in saunas or hot tubs, can reduce sperm count and motility. Similarly, exposure to low temperatures, such as in cold water or ice, can also have detrimental effects on male fertility [38].

Lifestyle Factors

Lifestyle factors refer to behaviors and habits that can contribute to male infertility [39]. These factors can be modified through lifestyle changes and can improve male reproductive function. Some of the most common lifestyle factors that have been linked to male infertility include diet, exercise, smoking, and alcohol consumption.

Diet

Diet can play a role in male fertility by providing essential nutrients and antioxidants that support healthy sperm production [39]. A diet that is high in processed foods, trans fats, and sugar has been linked to reduced sperm count and motility. Conversely, a diet that is rich in fruits, vegetables, and whole grains has been associated with improved sperm quality. Antioxidants such as vitamin C, vitamin E, and selenium have also been shown to improve sperm count and motility [40].

Exercise

Regular exercise can have a positive impact on male fertility by improving blood flow to the reproductive organs and reducing stress levels. However, excessive exercise or training can have the opposite effect and reduce sperm count and motility. Moderate exercise, such as brisk walking or cycling, is recommended to improve male fertility [41].

Smoking

Smoking is a known risk factor for male infertility. It can reduce sperm count and motility and increase the risk of DNA damage to sperm. Smoking can also affect the quality of semen by decreasing semen volume and altering the pH balance of the reproductive tract [42].

Alcohol Consumption

Excessive alcohol consumption can also have a negative impact on male fertility. It can reduce sperm count and motility and increase the risk of DNA damage to sperm. Alcohol can also affect the quality of semen by reducing semen volume and altering the pH balance of the reproductive tract [43].

Medical Conditions And Treatments

The causes of male infertility are multifactorial and can be divided into pre-testicular, testicular, and post-testicular factors. Medical conditions and treatments are among the post-testicular factors that can lead to male infertility. This chapter will discuss the medical conditions and treatments that can cause male infertility.

Medical Conditions

Varicocele: Varicocele is a medical condition characterized by enlarged veins within the scrotum. This condition affects 15% of men and is the most common cause of male infertility [44]. Varicocele can cause a decrease in sperm quality and quantity. The exact mechanism of how varicocele affects sperm production is still unclear. However, studies suggest that varicocele may cause oxidative stress and increase testicular temperature, which can affect sperm production [45].

Infections: Infections of the reproductive tract can lead to male infertility. Sexually transmitted infections such as chlamydia and gonorrhea can cause inflammation and scarring of the reproductive tract, leading to the obstruction of the sperm pathway [46, 47]. Other infections, such as mumps, tuberculosis, and prostatitis, can also affect sperm production and quality [48].

Hormonal Imbalances: Hormonal imbalances can also cause male infertility. The hypothalamic-pituitary-gonadal axis regulates the production of testosterone and sperm [16]. Any disruption in this axis can lead to hormonal imbalances that affect sperm production. Medical conditions such as hypogonadism, hyperprolactinemia, and thyroid disorders can affect the hormonal balance and lead to male infertility [27].

Retrograde Ejaculation: Retrograde ejaculation is a medical condition where semen is ejaculated into the bladder instead of out through the penis. This condition can occur due to nerve damage, medications, or surgery. Retrograde ejaculation can cause male infertility by reducing the number of sperm in the ejaculate [49].

Erectile Dysfunction: Erectile dysfunction is the inability to achieve or maintain an erection during sexual intercourse [50]. This condition can affect fertility by making it difficult for men to have sexual intercourse and ejaculate. Erectile dysfunction can be caused by medical conditions such as diabetes, hypertension, and cardiovascular disease [51].

Treatments

Chemotherapy: Chemotherapy is a treatment for cancer that uses drugs to kill cancer cells. Chemotherapy can cause male infertility by damaging the testicles and reducing sperm production. The risk of infertility depends on the type and dose of chemotherapy [52].

Radiation Therapy: Radiation therapy is another treatment for cancer that uses high-energy radiation to kill cancer cells. Radiation therapy can also affect sperm production by damaging the testicles. The risk of infertility depends on the dose and location of the radiation [37].

Surgery: Surgery can also cause male infertility. Surgical procedures such as vasectomy and varicocelectomy can lead to obstruction of the sperm pathway and reduce sperm production. In some cases, surgery can also cause nerve damage that leads to retrograde ejaculation [44, 45].

Medications: Some medications can affect sperm production and quality. Medications such as anabolic steroids, antipsychotics, and antidepressants can affect the hormonal balance and reduce sperm production [53]. Chemotherapeutic drugs used to treat autoimmune diseases, such as methotrexate and cyclophosphamide, can also affect sperm production [52].

Immunotherapy: Immunotherapy is a treatment for cancer that uses the immune system of the body to fight cancer cells [53]. Immunotherapy can cause male infertility by damaging the testicles and reducing sperm production. The risk of infertility depends on the type and dose of immunotherapy [54].

PSYCHOLOGICAL IMPACT OF MALE INFERTILITY

The psychological impact of infertility on men is often overlooked, and it can result in emotional distress, anxiety, and depression [55]. This chapter focuses on the psychological impact of male infertility, coping strategies, and the importance of seeking support.

Emotional Distress

Male infertility is associated with psychological distress that affects the mental health of a man, interpersonal relationships, and overall quality of life [56]. Men with infertility often experience feelings of guilt, shame, and inadequacy, leading to a loss of self-esteem and self-confidence [57]. These feelings can result in depression, anxiety, and stress.

Depression is a common mental health problem among infertile men [55]. In a study conducted by Peterson and colleagues (2003), it was found that men with infertility had higher rates of depression than men without infertility [58]. Depression is a serious mental health condition that can lead to a lack of motivation, loss of interest in activities, and suicidal ideation [55, 59]. Furthermore, anxiety is also a prevalent problem among infertile men. Anxiety is characterized by excessive worry and fear that can interfere with daily activities [60]. Men with infertility often worry about their ability to father a child, the effectiveness of treatments, and the financial cost of fertility treatments [61].

Stress is also a significant problem among men with infertility [62]. Infertility-related stress is caused by various factors such as the time and effort required for fertility treatments, financial burden, and fear of failure [55, 62]. Stress can have a negative impact on the physical health, mental health, and overall well-being of a man [56].

Anger and Frustration: Infertility can also cause men to experience anger and frustration. A study by Peterson and colleagues (2003) found that men with infertility experience more intense anger than their female partners. This anger can be directed toward themselves, their partners, and medical professionals, leading to strained relationships and increased stress [58].

Low Self-Esteem: Male infertility can lead to a decrease in self-esteem and self-worth. Men may feel inadequate, less masculine, or like they are not fulfilling their societal roles. A study by Daniluk and Koert (2008) found that men with infertility report lower self-esteem and feel less in control of their lives.

Coping Strategies

Coping strategies refer to the psychological mechanisms that individuals use to manage the stress associated with infertility. A study conducted by Peterson *et al.* (2011) found that coping strategies are important in determining the level of psychological distress experienced by infertile couples [63]. In general, coping strategies can be classified into two types: problem-focused coping and emotion-focused coping. Problem-focused coping strategies refer to efforts to actively address the problem that is causing stress, such as seeking medical treatment for infertility. In the context of male infertility, problem-focused coping strategies might include taking medication to improve sperm quality, undergoing surgery to correct a physical issue, or seeking the advice of a fertility specialist. Emotion-focused coping strategies, on the other hand, involve efforts to manage the emotional distress caused by the problem rather than trying to address the problem itself [64].

There are several emotion-focused coping strategies that can be used to manage the stress associated with male infertility. One such strategy is seeking social support. Research has shown that social support can be an important buffer against the negative psychological consequences of infertility [55]. Social support can come from a variety of sources, including family, friends, and support groups. Support groups can be particularly helpful because they provide a safe and supportive environment where individuals can share their experiences, express their feelings, and receive emotional support from others who are going through the same thing [65]. Another emotion-focused coping strategy is seeking professional help [66]. Infertility can be a very isolating experience, and sometimes, it can be difficult to talk to friends and family about what you are going through. A mental health professional, such as a therapist or counselor, can provide a safe and confidential space to talk about your feelings and work through the emotional challenges of infertility.

Self-care is another important coping strategy [67]. Infertility can be all-consuming, and it is easy to lose sight of your own needs and priorities. Taking care of yourself, both physically and emotionally, can help you manage the stress associated with infertility. This might include exercise, meditation, relaxation techniques, or engaging in hobbies or other activities that you enjoy [67]. Finally, reframing the situation can be an effective coping strategy. Reframing involves changing the way you think about a situation in order to reduce the stress it causes. In the context of male infertility, this might involve shifting your focus from the negative aspects of infertility to the positive aspects of your life. For example, you might focus on the things that you are grateful for, such as your relationship with your partner, your health, or your job [68].

Importance of Seeking Support

It is essential for men with infertility to seek support to manage the psychological impact of the condition. Support can be obtained from various sources, including family and friends, support groups, and mental health professionals.

Family and Friends

Family and friends can provide emotional support to men with infertility. A supportive partner can offer reassurance, love, and encouragement, which can help alleviate anxiety and depression. Supportive family and friends can also provide a listening ear and a shoulder to cry on, helping men cope with the negative emotions associated with infertility [59].

Support Groups

Infertility support groups can be a valuable source of support for men with infertility. Support groups provide a safe space for individuals to share their experiences, fears, and concerns with people who understand what they are going through. These groups offer a sense of community and belonging, which can help reduce feelings of isolation and loneliness [65].

Mental Health Professionals

Mental health professionals, such as therapists and psychologists, can provide specialized support to men with infertility [62]. They can help men manage their emotions, provide coping strategies, and assist with decision-making about fertility treatments. They can also help individuals work through issues that may be contributing to the psychological impact of infertility, such as relationship problems, stress, and anxiety [56].

FUTURE DIRECTIONS IN RESEARCH AND TREATMENT OF MALE INFERTILITY

Given the multifactorial nature of male infertility, future research endeavors are set to employ a multidimensional approach. Significant advancements in our understanding of male reproductive biology and the underlying causes of infertility may pave the way for the development of more effective treatment strategies.

Genomics and Epigenomics: The interplay between genetic and environmental factors can contribute to male infertility. Unraveling the complete spectrum of genetic variants and epigenetic modifications associated with male infertility remains a crucial area for future research. The use of next-generation sequencing technologies and genome-wide association studies (GWAS) can provide insights into potential genetic causes [69]. Epigenomic profiling, particularly the study of sperm DNA methylation and histone modifications, also holds promise in the identification of novel infertility markers [70].

Proteomics and Metabolomics: Proteomic and metabolomic analyses represent exciting avenues for future research, potentially revealing protein expression and metabolic alterations linked to male infertility [71]. These high-throughput technologies allow for an in-depth exploration of spermatozoal proteome and metabolome, potentially identifying unique biochemical signatures indicative of sperm health and fertility status [72].

Spermatogonial Stem Cells (SSCs) Therapy: SSCs hold the potential to treat various forms of male infertility, especially in cases of azoospermia [73]. Further research is required to optimize methods for SSC identification, isolation, expansion, and transplantation.

Assisted Reproductive Technologies (ART): With advances in ART, techniques such as intracytoplasmic sperm injection (ICSI), testicular sperm extraction (TESE), and *in-vitro* maturation (IVM) of sperm are poised for further optimization and development [59]. Advances in microfluidic sperm sorting technology also represent a significant development, potentially enhancing the selection of high-quality sperm for ART procedures [74].

Male Contraception: In the context of male fertility control, there is an unmet need for effective and reversible male contraceptives [75]. Future research should focus on the development of hormonal and non-hormonal male contraceptives, with an emphasis on ensuring reversibility and minimal side effects.

Lifestyle and Environmental Factors: More research is necessary to elucidate the impact of lifestyle factors (*e.g.*, diet, exercise, stress) and environmental toxins on male fertility. This could lead to more comprehensive fertility counseling and preventive strategies [39].

In conclusion, progress in male infertility research and treatment is dependent on integrative and innovative approaches, encompassing genomics, epigenomics, proteomics, metabolomics, SSCs therapy, advanced ART, male contraception, and lifestyle modification strategies. By pushing these frontiers, it is anticipated that more personalized and effective interventions for male infertility will be developed.

CONCLUSION

Male infertility, defined as the inability of a male to cause pregnancy in a fertile female, is a multifactorial condition that warrants thorough understanding for effective intervention. The male reproductive system is complex, encompassing several anatomical structures, each with specific functions. Hormonal regulation is crucial to the functioning of the male reproductive system. The causes of male infertility are diverse and can be grouped into genetic factors, environmental factors, lifestyle factors, and medical conditions/treatments. Genetic factors include chromosomal abnormalities and gene mutations, while environmental and lifestyle factors can range from exposure to toxins, smoking, alcohol consumption, and obesity to inadequate nutrition.

Certain medical conditions like varicocele, infections, hormonal imbalances, and treatments like chemotherapy and radiation can impair male fertility. The psychological impact of male infertility is significant, often leading to emotional distress. Coping strategies vary among individuals, underscoring the need for individualized mental health support.

There is a need to increase the recognition of the psychological implications of male infertility, encourage seeking mental health support, and ensure such resources are easily accessible and adequately equipped to handle the unique challenges associated with male infertility. Future research directions in the field of male infertility should focus on refining our understanding of its causes, improving diagnostic methods, developing novel treatments, and better addressing the psychological implications associated with this condition.

REFERENCES

[1]   Krausz C, Forti G. Clinical aspects of male infertility The genetic basis of male infertility. Berlin, Heidelberg: Springer 2000; pp. 1-21.

[2]   Barratt CLR, Björndahl L, De Jonge CJ, *et al.* The diagnosis of male infertility: an analysis of the evidence to support the development of global WHO guidance—challenges and future research opportunities. Hum Reprod Update 2017; 23(6): 660-80.
[http://dx.doi.org/10.1093/humupd/dmx021] [PMID: 28981651]

[3]   Infertility prevalence estimates: 1990–2021. World Helath Organization 2023.

[4]   Agarwal A, Mulgund A, Hamada A, Chyatte MR. A unique view on male infertility around the globe. Reprod Biol Endocrinol 2015; 13(1): 37.
[http://dx.doi.org/10.1186/s12958-015-0032-1] [PMID: 25928197]

[5]   Larsen U. Research on infertility: Which definition should we use? Fertil Steril 2005; 83(4): 846-52.
[http://dx.doi.org/10.1016/j.fertnstert.2004.11.033] [PMID: 15820788]

[6]   Olayemi F. Review on some causes of male infertility. Afr J Biotechnol 2010; 9.

[7]   Sengupta P, Dutta S, Krajewska-Kulak E. The disappearing sperms: analysis of reports published between 1980 and 2015. Am J Men Health 2017; 11(4): 1279-304.
[http://dx.doi.org/10.1177/1557988316643383] [PMID: 27099345]

[8]   Tournaye H. Male factor infertility and ART. Asian J Androl 2012; 14(1): 103-8.
[http://dx.doi.org/10.1038/aja.2011.65] [PMID: 22179511]

[9]   Aire TA. Anatomy of the testis and male reproductive tract. Reprod Biol Phyl Birds 2007; 6: 37-113.

[10]   Nieschlag E, Behre HM, Nieschlag S. Testosterone: action, deficiency, substitution. Cambridge University Press 2012.
[http://dx.doi.org/10.1017/CBO9781139003353]

[11]   Robaire B, Hinton BT, Orgebin-Crist M-C. The epididymis Knobil and Neill's physiology of reproduction. Elsevier 2006; pp. 1071-148.
[http://dx.doi.org/10.1016/B978-012515400-0/50027-0]

[12]   Koslov DS, Andersson KE. Physiological and pharmacological aspects of the vas deferens—an update. Front Pharmacol 2013; 4: 101.
[http://dx.doi.org/10.3389/fphar.2013.00101] [PMID: 23986701]

[13]   Aumüller G, Riva A. Morphology and functions of the human seminal vesicle. Andrologia 1992; 24(4): 183-96.
[http://dx.doi.org/10.1111/j.1439-0272.1992.tb02636.x] [PMID: 1642333]

[14]   McNeal JE. Normal histology of the prostate. Am J Surg Pathol 1988; 12(8): 619-33.
[http://dx.doi.org/10.1097/00000478-198808000-00003] [PMID: 2456702]

[15]   McCallum RW. The adult male urethra: normal anatomy, pathology, and method of urethrography. Radiol Clin North Am 1979; 17(2): 227-44.
[PMID: 472199]

[16]   Sengupta P, Arafa M, Elbardisi H. Hormonal regulation of spermatogenesis Molecular signaling in spermatogenesis and male infertility. CRC Press 2019; pp. 41-9.
[http://dx.doi.org/10.1201/9780429244216-5]

[17]   Nishimura H, L'Hernault SW. Spermatogenesis. Curr Biol 2017; 27(18): R988-94.
[http://dx.doi.org/10.1016/j.cub.2017.07.067] [PMID: 28950090]

[18]   O'Donnell L. Mechanisms of spermiogenesis and spermiation and how they are disturbed. Spermatogenesis 2014; 4(2): e979623.
[http://dx.doi.org/10.4161/21565562.2014.979623] [PMID: 26413397]

[19]   De Jonge C. Biological basis for human capacitation. Hum Reprod Update 2005; 11(3): 205-14.
[http://dx.doi.org/10.1093/humupd/dmi010] [PMID: 15817522]

[20]   Cross NL. Role of cholesterol in sperm capacitation. Biol Reprod 1998; 59(1): 7-11.
[http://dx.doi.org/10.1095/biolreprod59.1.7] [PMID: 9674986]

[21]   Russell LD, Saxena NK, Turner TT. Cytoskeletal involvement in spermiation and sperm transport. Tissue Cell 1989; 21(3): 361-79.
[http://dx.doi.org/10.1016/0040-8166(89)90051-7] [PMID: 2479117]

[22]   Jaiswal BS, Eisenbach M. Capacitation Fertilization. Elsevier 2002; pp. 57-117.
[http://dx.doi.org/10.1016/B978-012311629-1/50005-X]

[23]   Visconti PE, Kopf GS. Regulation of protein phosphorylation during sperm capacitation. Biol Reprod 1998; 59(1): 1-6.
[http://dx.doi.org/10.1095/biolreprod59.1.1] [PMID: 9674985]

[24] Breitbart H, Naor Z. Protein kinases in mammalian sperm capacitation and the acrosome reaction. Rev Reprod 1999; 4(3): 151-9.
[http://dx.doi.org/10.1530/ror.0.0040151] [PMID: 10521152]

[25] Miller WL, Auchus RJ. The molecular biology, biochemistry, and physiology of human steroidogenesis and its disorders. Endocr Rev 2011; 32(1): 81-151.
[http://dx.doi.org/10.1210/er.2010-0013] [PMID: 21051590]

[26] Mindnich R, Möller G, Adamski J. The role of 17 beta-hydroxysteroid dehydrogenases. Mol Cell Endocrinol 2004; 218(1-2): 7-20.
[http://dx.doi.org/10.1016/j.mce.2003.12.006] [PMID: 15130507]

[27] Dutta S, Sengupta P, Muhamad S. Male reproductive hormones and semen quality. Asian Pac J Reprod 2019; 8(5): 189-94.
[http://dx.doi.org/10.4103/2305-0500.268132]

[28] Ferlin A, Arredi B, Foresta C. Genetic causes of male infertility. Reprod Toxicol 2006; 22(2): 133-41.
[http://dx.doi.org/10.1016/j.reprotox.2006.04.016] [PMID: 16806807]

[29] Krausz C, Riera-Escamilla A. Genetics of male infertility. Nat Rev Urol 2018; 15(6): 369-84.
[http://dx.doi.org/10.1038/s41585-018-0003-3] [PMID: 29622783]

[30] Harton GL, Tempest HG. Chromosomal disorders and male infertility. Asian J Androl 2012; 14(1): 32-9.
[http://dx.doi.org/10.1038/aja.2011.66] [PMID: 22120929]

[31] Cuppens H, Cassiman JJ. CFTR mutations and polymorphisms in male infertility. Int J Androl 2004; 27(5): 251-6.
[http://dx.doi.org/10.1111/j.1365-2605.2004.00485.x] [PMID: 15379964]

[32] Hiort O, Holterhus PM. Androgen insensitivity and male infertility. Int J Androl 2003; 26(1): 16-20.
[http://dx.doi.org/10.1046/j.1365-2605.2003.00369.x] [PMID: 12534933]

[33] Okada H, Fujioka H, Tatsumi N, *et al.* Klinefelter's syndrome in the male infertility clinic. Hum Reprod 1999; 14(4): 946-52.
[http://dx.doi.org/10.1093/humrep/14.4.946] [PMID: 10221225]

[34] Sengupta P. Environmental and occupational exposure of metals and their role in male reproductive functions. Drug Chem Toxicol 2013; 36(3): 353-68.
[http://dx.doi.org/10.3109/01480545.2012.710631] [PMID: 22947100]

[35] Sengupta P, Banerjee R. Environmental toxins. Hum Exp Toxicol 2014; 33(10): 1017-39.
[http://dx.doi.org/10.1177/0960327113515504] [PMID: 24347299]

[36] Dutta S, Sengupta P, Bagchi S, *et al.* Reproductive toxicity of combined effects of endocrine disruptors on human reproduction. Front Cell Dev Biol 2023; 11: 1162015.
[http://dx.doi.org/10.3389/fcell.2023.1162015] [PMID: 37250900]

[37] Kesari KK, Agarwal A, Henkel R. Radiations and male fertility. Reprod Biol Endocrinol 2018; 16(1): 118.
[http://dx.doi.org/10.1186/s12958-018-0431-1] [PMID: 30445985]

[38] Al-Otaibi ST. Male infertility among bakers associated with exposure to high environmental temperature at the workplace. J Taibah Univ Med Sci 2018; 13(2): 103-7.
[http://dx.doi.org/10.1016/j.jtumed.2017.12.003] [PMID: 31435311]

[39] Durairajanayagam D. Lifestyle causes of male infertility. Arab J Urol 2018; 16(1): 10-20.
[http://dx.doi.org/10.1016/j.aju.2017.12.004] [PMID: 29713532]

[40] Sinclair S. Male infertility: nutritional and environmental considerations. Altern Med Rev 2000; 5(1): 28-38.
[PMID: 10696117]

[41]   Arce JC, De Souza MJ. Exercise and male factor infertility. Sports Med 1993; 15(3): 146-69.
       [http://dx.doi.org/10.2165/00007256-199315030-00002] [PMID: 8451548]

[42]   Harlev A, Agarwal A, Gunes SO, Shetty A, du Plessis SS. Smoking and male infertility: an evidence-
       based review. World J Mens Health 2015; 33(3): 143-60.
       [http://dx.doi.org/10.5534/wjmh.2015.33.3.143] [PMID: 26770934]

[43]   La Vignera S, Condorelli RA, Balercia G, Vicari E, Calogero AE. Does alcohol have any effect on
       male reproductive function? A review of literature. Asian J Androl 2013; 15(2): 221-5.
       [http://dx.doi.org/10.1038/aja.2012.118] [PMID: 23274392]

[44]   Agarwal A, Finelli R, Durairajanayagam D, *et al.* Comprehensive analysis of global research on
       human varicocele: a scientometric approach. World J Mens Health 2022; 40(4): 636-52.
       [http://dx.doi.org/10.5534/wjmh.210202] [PMID: 35118839]

[45]   Jensen CFS, Østergren P, Dupree JM, Ohl DA, Sønksen J, Fode M. Varicocele and male infertility.
       Nat Rev Urol 2017; 14(9): 523-33.
       [http://dx.doi.org/10.1038/nrurol.2017.98] [PMID: 28675168]

[46]   Dutta S, Sengupta P, Chhikara BS. Reproductive inflammatory mediators and male infertility. Chem
       Biol Lett 2020; 7: 73-4.

[47]   Dutta S, Sengupta P, Slama P, Roychoudhury S. Oxidative stress, testicular inflammatory pathways,
       and male reproduction. Int J Mol Sci 2021; 22(18): 10043.
       [http://dx.doi.org/10.3390/ijms221810043] [PMID: 34576205]

[48]   Sengupta P, Dutta S, Alahmar AT. Reproductive tract infection, inflammation and male infertility.
       Chem Biol Lett 2020; 7: 75-84.

[49]   Gupta S, Sharma R, Agarwal A, *et al.* A comprehensive guide to sperm recovery in infertile men with
       retrograde ejaculation. World J Mens Health 2022; 40(2): 208-16.
       [http://dx.doi.org/10.5534/wjmh.210069] [PMID: 34169680]

[50]   Kessler A, Sollie S, Challacombe B, Briggs K, Van Hemelrijck M. The global prevalence of erectile
       dysfunction: a review. BJU Int 2019; 124(4): 587-99.
       [http://dx.doi.org/10.1111/bju.14813] [PMID: 31267639]

[51]   McMahon CG. Current diagnosis and management of erectile dysfunction. Med J Aust 2019; 210(10):
       469-76.
       [http://dx.doi.org/10.5694/mja2.50167] [PMID: 31099420]

[52]   Schrader M, Heicappell R, Müller M, Straub B, Miller K. Impact of chemotherapy on male fertility.
       Onkologie 2001; 24(4): 326-30.
       [PMID: 11574759]

[53]   Izuka E, Menuba I, Sengupta P, Dutta S, Nwagha U. Antioxidants, anti-inflammatory drugs and
       antibiotics in the treatment of reproductive tract infections and their association with male infertility.
       Chem Biol Lett 2020; 7: 156-65.

[54]   O'Donnell L, Smith LB, Rebourcet D. Sperm-specific proteins: new implications for diagnostic
       development and cancer immunotherapy. Curr Opin Cell Biol 2022; 77: 102104.
       [http://dx.doi.org/10.1016/j.ceb.2022.102104] [PMID: 35671587]

[55]   Kedem P, Mikulincer M, Nathanson YE, Bartoov B. Psychological aspects of male infertility. Br J
       Med Psychol 1990; 63(1): 73-80.
       [http://dx.doi.org/10.1111/j.2044-8341.1990.tb02858.x] [PMID: 2331455]

[56]   Dong M, Wu S, Zhang X, Zhao N, Tao Y, Tan J. Impact of infertility duration on male sexual function
       and mental health. J Assist Reprod Genet 2022; 39(8): 1861-72.
       [http://dx.doi.org/10.1007/s10815-022-02550-9] [PMID: 35838818]

[57]   Xing X, Pan B-C, Du Q, Liang X, Wang X-M, Wang L. [Impact of male infertility on men's self-
       esteem and satisfaction with sexual relationship]. Zhonghua Nan Ke Xue 2013; 19(3): 223-7.

[PMID: 23700727]

[58]   Peterson BD, Newton CR, Rosen KH. Examining congruence between partners' perceived infertility-related stress and its relationship to marital adjustment and depression in infertile couples. Fam Process 2003; 42(1): 59-70.
[http://dx.doi.org/10.1111/j.1545-5300.2003.00059.x] [PMID: 12698599]

[59]   Daar AS, Merali Z. Infertility and social suffering: the case of ART in developing countries. Current practices and controversies in assisted reproduction. World Health Organization, Geneva 2002;15:21

[60]   Öztekin Ü, Hacimusalar Y, Gürel A, Karaaslan O. The relationship of male infertility with somatosensory amplification, health anxiety and depression levels. Psychiatry Investig 2020; 17(4): 350-5.
[http://dx.doi.org/10.30773/pi.2019.0248] [PMID: 32252512]

[61]   Leung AK, Henry MA, Mehta A. Gaps in male infertility health services research. Transl Androl Urol 2018; 7(S3) (Suppl. 3): S303-9.
[http://dx.doi.org/10.21037/tau.2018.05.03] [PMID: 30159236]

[62]   Basu S. Psychological stress and male infertility Male Infertility: A Complete Guide to Lifestyle and Environmental Factors. Springer 2014; pp. 141-59.

[63]   Peterson BD, Pirritano M, Block JM, Schmidt L. Marital benefit and coping strategies in men and women undergoing unsuccessful fertility treatments over a 5-year period. Fertil Steril 2011; 95: 1759-63.

[64]   Levin JB, Sher TG, Theodos V. The effect of intracouple coping concordance on psychological and marital distress in infertility patients. J Clin Psychol Med Settings 1997; 4(4): 361-72.
[http://dx.doi.org/10.1023/A:1026249317635]

[65]   Martins MV, Peterson BD, Almeida V, Mesquita-Guimarães J, Costa ME. Dyadic dynamics of perceived social support in couples facing infertility. Hum Reprod 2014; 29(1): 83-9.
[http://dx.doi.org/10.1093/humrep/det403] [PMID: 24218401]

[66]   Malik SH, Coulson N. The male experience of infertility: a thematic analysis of an online infertility support group bulletin board. J Reprod Infant Psychol 2008; 26(1): 18-30.
[http://dx.doi.org/10.1080/02646830701759777]

[67]   Blenner JL. Attaining self-care in infertility treatment. Appl Nurs Res 1990; 3(3): 98-104.
[http://dx.doi.org/10.1016/S0897-1897(05)80124-7] [PMID: 2400214]

[68]   Zucker DJ, Benjamin A. He said/She said; Shaming, Blaming … Reframing: Impacts and Implications of Childlessness on Relationships in an Ancient Text. J Pastoral Care Counsel 2020; 74(3): 182-8.
[http://dx.doi.org/10.1177/1542305020924997] [PMID: 32967541]

[69]   Salvi R, Gawde U, Idicula-Thomas S, Biswas B. Pathway Analysis of Genome Wide Association Studies (GWAS) Data Associated with Male Infertility. Reproductive Medicine 2022; 3(3): 235-45.
[http://dx.doi.org/10.3390/reprodmed3030018]

[70]   Darbandi M, Darbandi S, Agarwal A, *et al.* Reactive oxygen species-induced alterations in H19-Igf2 methylation patterns, seminal plasma metabolites, and semen quality. J Assist Reprod Genet 2019; 36(2): 241-53.
[http://dx.doi.org/10.1007/s10815-018-1350-y] [PMID: 30382470]

[71]   Jodar M, Soler-Ventura A, Oliva R. Semen proteomics and male infertility. J Proteomics 2017; 162: 125-34.
[http://dx.doi.org/10.1016/j.jprot.2016.08.018] [PMID: 27576136]

[72]   Minai-Tehrani A, Jafarzadeh N, Gilany K. Metabolomics: a state-of-the-art technology for better understanding of male infertility. Andrologia 2016; 48(6): 609-16.
[http://dx.doi.org/10.1111/and.12496] [PMID: 26608970]

[73]   Zarandi NP, Galdon G, Kogan S, Atala A, Sadri-Ardekani H. Cryostorage of immature and mature

human testis tissue to preserve spermatogonial stem cells (SSCs): a systematic review of current experiences toward clinical applications. Stem Cells Cloning Adv Appl 2018; pp. 23-38.

[74]   Samuel R, Feng H, Jafek A, Despain D, Jenkins T, Gale B. Microfluidic—based sperm sorting & analysis for treatment of male infertility. Transl Androl Urol 2018; 7(S3) (Suppl. 3): S336-47.
[http://dx.doi.org/10.21037/tau.2018.05.08] [PMID: 30159240]

[75]   Amory JK. Male contraception. Fertil Steril 2016; 106(6): 1303-9.
[http://dx.doi.org/10.1016/j.fertnstert.2016.08.036] [PMID: 27678037]

CHAPTER 2

Molecular Mechanism of Male Infertility

Abstract: Male infertility is a significant global health concern, necessitating an understanding of its molecular basis to develop effective diagnostics and treatments. Spermatogenesis is pivotal to fertility, the process within the testes that produces mature spermatozoa capable of fertilizing oocytes. Additionally, sperm maturation, which occurs in the male reproductive tract, includes pre-capacitation and capacitation stages, both critical for fertilization. Male infertility can result from disruptions in these processes due to factors such as genetic mutations, impaired sperm motility, hormonal imbalances, and oxidative stress (OS). Genetic alterations can affect genes crucial for spermatogenesis, sperm function, or hormonal regulation. Reduced sperm motility hampers the ability of sperm to reach the oocyte, while hormonal imbalances disrupt the optimal environment for sperm production. OS, arising from an imbalance between reactive oxygen species (ROS) and antioxidants, can cause sperm DNA damage. Cutting-edge research in genomics and epigenomics provides insights into the genetic factors of infertility. Single-cell genomics enables the analysis of individual sperm cells, contributing to a detailed understanding of genetic variation. Furthermore, investigating environmental and lifestyle factors sheds light on their impact on male fertility. Advanced assisted reproductive technologies (ART) and precision medicine, which tailor treatment based on individual genetics and physiology, offer promising solutions for affected couples. The present chapter aims to elucidate the intricate molecular mechanisms underlying male infertility, encompassing genetic, cellular, and endocrine components, and sheds light on future perspectives of in-depth diagnostic and therapeutic interventions. Ongoing research is pivotal for developing targeted interventions and improving reproductive health outcomes.

Keywords: Andrology, Assisted Reproductive Techniques, Azoospermia, DNA Damage, Epididymis, Epigenetics, Gonadotropins, Infertility, Male Urogenital Diseases, Oligospermia, Oxidative Stress, Sertoli Cells, Sperm Count, Sperm Motility, Spermatozoa, Spermatogenesis, Spermatogonia, Testosterone, Varicocele, Y-Chromosome Infertility.

INTRODUCTION

Male infertility is a condition where a man is unable to impregnate a woman despite having unprotected sexual intercourse for a year or more. Infertility affects approximately 15% of couples worldwide, and male factors contribute to approximately 50% of cases [1]. Male infertility can be caused by various factors, including genetic, environmental, and lifestyle factors [2]. Some common causes of male infertility include low sperm count, poor sperm motility, abnormal sperm shape, and problems with ejaculation [3, 4].

Infertility is a significant public health issue with significant medical, emotional, and economic consequences [5, 6]. It affects millions of couples worldwide, and male infertility is a critical factor in about half of infertility cases [1, 7]. Understanding the molecular mechanisms underlying male infertility can help identify the causes of infertility and provide a basis for developing effective treatments. Recent advances in molecular biology and genomics have provided new insights into the molecular mechanisms underlying male infertility [8]. These advances have led to the identification of numerous genes and molecular pathways that are involved in sperm production, maturation, and function. Understanding the molecular basis of male infertility can provide new targets for the development of diagnostic tools and therapies for infertility [8, 9]. In this chapter, we will review the molecular mechanisms underlying male infertility and discuss recent advances in the field.

CAUSES OF MALE INFERTILITY

As discussed in detail in Chapter 1, male infertility, a multifactorial condition affecting reproductive capability in males, can be caused by various genetic, environmental, and lifestyle factors [2].

Genetic factors include chromosomal abnormalities, gene mutations, and epigenetic changes. Klinefelter syndrome, a chromosomal anomaly causing an extra X chromosome, leads to testicular atrophy and reduced testosterone levels, thus infertility. Y chromosome microdeletions also contribute to infertility due to the loss of key genes required for male fertility [10, 11]. Gene mutations affecting spermatogenesis, such as those in the CFTR and FSH receptor genes, can lead to abnormal sperm production and function. Epigenetic factors, like DNA methylation and histone modifications, can alter gene expression, thereby influencing spermatogenesis. Methylation of the H19 gene, for instance, can cause infertility if disrupted. Other potential factors encompass exposure to harmful chemicals, lifestyle choices, and occupation [12]. Pesticides, like organophosphates, carbamates, and pyrethroids, impair spermatogenesis and other sperm characteristics, leading to infertility. Heavy metals, such as lead, cadmium, and mercury, can accumulate in the body and cause damage to the testicular cells, disrupting spermatogenesis [13, 14]. Lifestyle factors, including smoking, alcohol consumption, and obesity, adversely affect male fertility, with each causing a variety of hormonal imbalances and sperm abnormalities [15]. Lastly, occupational exposure to various chemicals can have detrimental effects on male fertility, particularly in industries like agriculture, chemical production, and metallurgy [14] (*Refer to* Chapter 1).

MOLECULAR MECHANISMS OF MALE INFERTILITY

Gene Mutations

Genetic causes of male infertility are associated with mutations in genes involved in spermatogenesis, sperm motility, and hormonal regulation [16] Fig. (**4**).

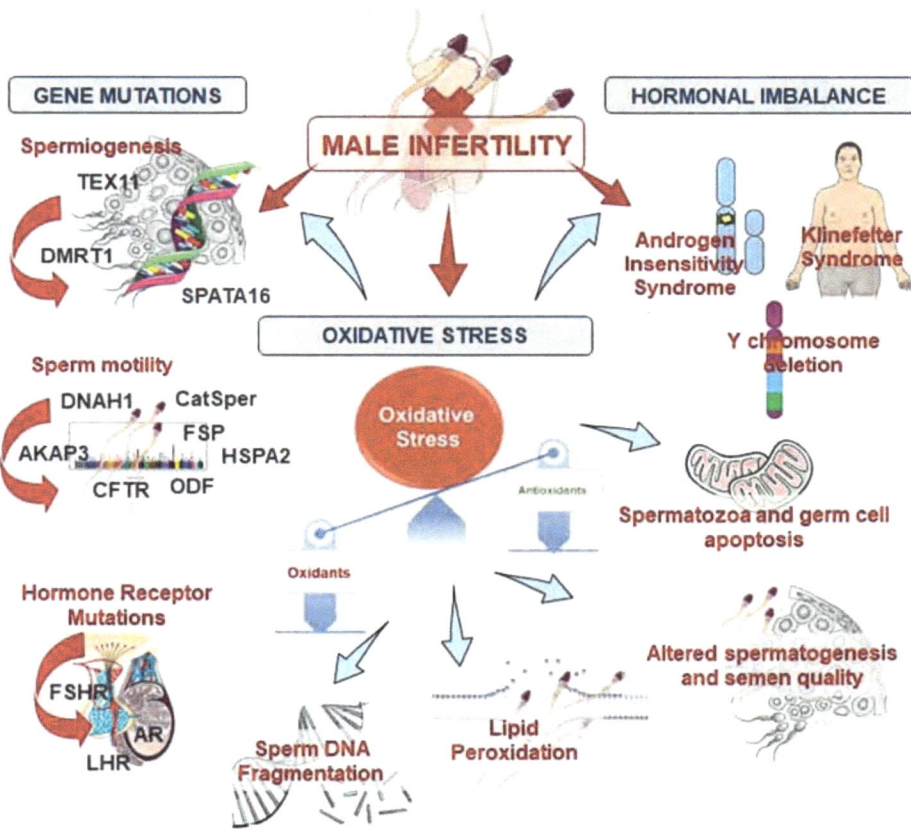

Fig. (4). Molecular mechanisms of male infertility. These include gene mutations of spermatogenesis, hormone receptors, hormonal imbalances, and oxidative stress.

Spermatogenesis

Spermatogenesis is the process of sperm cell development from spermatogonia to mature spermatozoa. It is a complex and highly regulated process that involves several genes. Mutations in these genes can result in impaired spermatogenesis and male infertility. Some of the genes involved in spermatogenesis are:

TEX11: TEX11 is a testis-specific gene that is essential for spermatogenesis. Mutations in TEX11 are associated with impaired spermatogenesis and male infertility [17]. TEX11 is involved in the formation of synaptonemal complexes during meiosis, which are essential for homologous recombination and segregation of chromosomes. TEX11 mutations result in meiotic arrest and failure to progress beyond the pachytene stage of meiosis [18].

DMRT1: DMRT1 is a transcription factor that is essential for testis development and spermatogenesis [19]. Mutations in DMRT1 are associated with impaired spermatogenesis and male infertility. DMRT1 is involved in the regulation of gene expression during spermatogenesis and is essential for the maintenance of germ cells. DMRT1 mutations result in a decrease in the number of germ cells and impaired spermatogenesis [20].

SPATA16: SPATA16 is a gene that is essential for spermatogenesis. Mutations in SPATA16 are associated with impaired spermatogenesis and male infertility [21]. SPATA16 is involved in the regulation of meiotic recombination and is essential for the proper segregation of chromosomes during meiosis. SPATA16 mutations result in meiotic arrest and failure to progress beyond the pachytene stage of meiosis [22].

Sperm Motility

Sperm motility is essential for fertilization, and mutations in genes involved in sperm motility can result in male infertility. Some of the genes involved in sperm motility are:

DNAH1: Dynein axonemal heavy chain 1 (DNAH1) is a gene that encodes a dynein protein that is essential for ciliary and flagellar motility [23]. Mutations in DNAH1 are associated with impaired sperm motility and male infertility. DNAH1 mutations result in the absence of dynein arms in the sperm flagellum, which impairs the movement of sperm [24].

AKAP3: AKAP3 is a gene that encodes a protein that is involved in the regulation of sperm motility. Mutations in AKAP3 are associated with impaired sperm motility and male infertility [25]. AKAP3 is involved in the regulation of protein kinase A (PKA), which is essential for the regulation of sperm motility. AKAP3 mutations result in impaired PKA regulation and impaired sperm motility [26].

CFTR: CFTR is a gene that encodes a chloride channel that is essential for the regulation of fluid and electrolyte transport in the male reproductive system. Mutations in CFTR are associated with impaired sperm motility and male infertility [16]. CFTR mutations result in the absence or dysfunction of the chloride channel, which impairs the regulation of fluid and electrolyte transport in the male reproductive system [10].

Hormonal Regulations

Hormonal regulation is critical for male fertility, as it controls the production of sperm and other reproductive functions [27]. Testosterone, follicle-stimulating hormone (FSH), and luteinizing hormone (LH) are the three most important hormones involved in male fertility. Testosterone is produced in the testes and is responsible for the development of male characteristics, such as facial hair and a deep voice. FSH and LH are produced in the pituitary gland and stimulate the testes to produce sperm [28]. There are a variety of gene mutations that can contribute to hormonal regulation and cause male infertility [29]. Some of these mutations affect the genes that are involved in the production of hormones, while others affect the genes that are responsible for the receptors that receive the hormones. Mutations can occur spontaneously or be inherited from parents [30]. One of the most common gene mutations associated with male infertility is a mutation in the FSH receptor gene. This gene is responsible for producing the receptor that receives FSH and stimulates the production of sperm. Mutations in this gene can result in a decrease in the production of sperm and contribute to male infertility [31]. Another important gene mutation associated with male infertility is a mutation in the androgen receptor gene. This gene is responsible for producing the receptor that receives testosterone and is critical for the development of male characteristics. Mutations in this gene can result in a decrease in the production of testosterone and contribute to male infertility [32]. Other gene mutations associated with male infertility include mutations in the LH receptor gene, the inhibin alpha gene, and the estrogen receptor gene. All of these genes are critical for hormonal regulation and can contribute to male infertility when they are mutated [33].

Abnormal Sperm Motility

Sperm motility is an essential aspect of male fertility, and its dysfunction can lead to infertility in men [34]. Several factors can contribute to abnormal sperm motility, including genetic mutations. Gene mutations causing abnormal sperm motility can occur at various levels, including gene expression, protein structure, and regulation. These mutations can result in a wide range of phenotypes, including reduced motility, abnormal morphology, and inability to fertilize the egg [35]. This write-up will discuss some of the common gene mutations causing abnormal sperm motility.

Dynein Axonemal Heavy Chain (DNAH) Mutations

DNAH is a protein that plays a crucial role in sperm motility by powering the movement of cilia and flagella [23]. DNAH mutations are associated with primary ciliary dyskinesia (PCD), a rare autosomal recessive disorder characterized by abnormal cilia and flagella function. PCD affects approximately 1 in 15,000 individuals, and up to 50% of male PCD patients experience infertility due to reduced or absent sperm motility [36]. DNAH mutations account for up to 30% of cases of PCD-associated infertility. A study of 113 PCD patients with infertility found that DNAH11 mutations were the most common cause of infertility, accounting for 24% of cases [24].

Catsper Channel Mutations

The Catsper channel is a calcium ion channel located on the surface of sperm cells that plays a crucial role in sperm motility and fertilization [37]. Mutations in Catsper genes can lead to reduced sperm motility and male infertility [38]. Catsper mutations are rare, with only a few reported cases in the literature. However, a recent study of a consanguineous family with three infertile male siblings identified a homozygous missense mutation in Catsper1 that resulted in abnormal sperm motility [39].

Fibrous Sheath Protein (FSP) Mutations

FSP are structural proteins that provide support to the axoneme and play a crucial role in sperm motility [40]. FSP mutations can lead to reduced or absent sperm motility and male infertility. A study of 40 infertile men with abnormal sperm motility identified FSP1 mutations in 7.5% of cases [41].

Outer Dense Fiber (ODF) Mutations

ODF are structural proteins that provide support to the sperm tail and play a role in sperm motility [36]. ODF mutations can lead to reduced or absent sperm motility and male infertility. A study of 17 infertile men with asthenozoospermia identified ODF1 mutations in two of the patients [42].

Heat Shock Protein A2 (HSPA2) Mutations

Heat shock protein A2 (HSPA2) is a chaperone protein that plays a crucial role in spermatogenesis and sperm function. HSPA2 mutations are associated with reduced sperm motility and male infertility.

Hormonal Imbalances

Hormonal imbalances in males can have various causes, including genetic and environmental factors [43]. Hormones are chemical messengers that are produced by the endocrine glands, and they play a crucial role in regulating various bodily functions, including reproduction. In males, testosterone is the primary sex hormone that is responsible for the development of male sexual characteristics and sperm production [28]. Any disruption in the production or regulation of testosterone can result in hormonal imbalances, which can, in turn, lead to male infertility [43, 44].

Androgen Insensitivity Syndrome (AIS)

AIS is a genetic condition that affects the development of male sexual characteristics [45]. It is caused by mutations in the androgen receptor (AR) gene, which codes for a protein that is essential for the function of testosterone. The AR protein is a transcription factor that binds to testosterone and regulates the expression of target genes. In individuals with AIS, the AR protein is dysfunctional, and it cannot bind to testosterone, resulting in a lack of male sexual development [32]. AIS is classified into three types based on the severity of the condition. In complete AIS, the AR protein is entirely dysfunctional, and affected individuals have female external genitalia and internal testes. In partial AIS, the AR protein is partially functional, resulting in ambiguous genitalia and incomplete male sexual development. In mild AIS, the AR protein is slightly dysfunctional, and affected individuals have male external genitalia but may have breast development [32, 45].

Klinefelter Syndrome

Klinefelter syndrome is a genetic condition that affects males, and it is caused by an extra copy of the X chromosome [11]. Most males have one X and one Y chromosome, but individuals with Klinefelter syndrome have two X chromosomes and one Y chromosome (47, XXY). This extra chromosome results in the production of less testosterone than normal, leading to hormonal imbalances and male infertility. Individuals with Klinefelter syndrome may have a range of physical and developmental symptoms, including small testes, gynecomastia (breast development), reduced muscle mass, and decreased body hair. They may also have learning disabilities and behavioral problems [10, 11].

Y Chromosome Deletions

The Y chromosome is the sex chromosome that is responsible for the development of male sexual characteristics. It contains genes that code for various proteins, including the sex-determining region Y (SRY) gene, which initiates male sexual development [46]. Deletions in the Y chromosome can result in the loss of critical genes that are essential for male reproductive function, leading to hormonal imbalances and male infertility. Y chromosome deletions are one of the most common genetic causes of male infertility, and they occur in approximately 7% of infertile males. The severity of the condition depends on the size and location of the deletion. Some deletions may have no effect on male reproductive function, while others may result in complete azoospermia (no sperm production) [46, 47].

Types of Hormone Receptor Mutations

Hormone receptor mutations can affect different types of receptors in the male reproductive system. The most common types of hormone receptors involved in male fertility are the androgen receptor (AR) and the follicle-stimulating hormone receptor (FSHR) [31, 32].

Androgen Receptor Mutations: The androgen receptor is a protein that is found in the cytoplasm of cells in the male reproductive system. It plays a critical role in the development and maintenance of male sexual characteristics, including the growth of facial hair, deepening of the voice, and development of the testes [28]. Androgens, such as testosterone, bind to the androgen receptor, triggering a cascade of cellular responses that regulate male sexual development and function. Mutations in the androgen receptor gene can lead to a wide range of AIS, a group of genetic disorders characterized by varying degrees of feminization of male genitalia and infertility. The severity of the disorder depends on the type and location of the mutation. Complete androgen insensitivity syndrome (CAIS) is the most severe form of AIS and is characterized by a complete lack of androgen receptor function. Individuals with CAIS have a female phenotype and do not develop male genitalia. Partial androgen insensitivity syndrome (PAIS) is a milder form of AIS, where individuals have some androgen receptor function but with varying degrees of feminization and infertility. In mild forms of PAIS, individuals may have a male phenotype but may still exhibit some degree of infertility [28, 45].

FSH Receptor Mutations: The follicle-stimulating hormone receptor is a protein that is found on the surface of cells in the testes. It plays a critical role in the development and maturation of sperm cells. FSH binds to the receptor, stimulating the production of sperm cells. Mutations in the FSH receptor gene can lead to a variety of disorders, including hypogonadotropic hypogonadism (HH) and idiopathic infertility [31]. HH is a condition where the testes do not produce enough testosterone, leading to infertility and other symptoms. Idiopathic infertility is a condition where the cause of infertility is unknown.

Oxidative Stress

While the causes of infertility can be numerous, one factor that has gained attention in recent years is oxidative stress. Oxidative stress is a state where there is an imbalance between the production of reactive oxygen species (ROS) and the ability of the body to neutralize them. It has been suggested that oxidative stress can be a contributing factor to male infertility [48]. Oxidative stress is a state where there is an imbalance between the production of ROS and the ability of the body to neutralize them. Reactive oxygen species are chemically reactive molecules that can cause damage to cellular structures, including lipids, proteins, and DNA. Normally, the body can neutralize ROS through the use of antioxidants, which can either prevent the production of ROS or neutralize them before they can cause damage. However, when there is an excess production of ROS or a deficiency in antioxidant defenses, oxidative stress can occur. Oxidative stress has been implicated in numerous disease states, including cancer, cardiovascular disease, and neurodegenerative diseases [49]. Oxidative stress has been suggested as a possible cause of male infertility. The testes are particularly vulnerable to oxidative stress due to their high metabolic activity and the presence of unsaturated fatty acids in the sperm cell membranes, which are susceptible to ROS damage. ROS can cause damage to sperm DNA, leading to genetic abnormalities that can affect fertility. ROS can also damage the sperm cell membrane, leading to decreased motility and viability. In addition, ROS can lead to an increase in white blood cells in semen, which can further contribute to oxidative stress [18, 50].

Causes of Oxidative Stress in Male Infertility

There are several factors that can contribute to oxidative stress in male infertility. One of the most significant factors is lifestyle. Habits such as smoking, excessive alcohol consumption, and drug use can all contribute to oxidative stress [15]. In addition, exposure to environmental toxins, such as heavy metals and pesticides, can also contribute to oxidative stress [13]. Other causes of oxidative stress in male infertility include infections, varicoceles, and age [2, 51]. Infections can cause an increase in white blood cells in semen, which can lead to oxidative stress [52]. Varicoceles are enlarged veins in the scrotum that can lead to increased testicular temperature and oxidative stress [51]. Finally, as men age, there is a decrease in antioxidant defenses, which can lead to an increase in oxidative stress [2].

Effects of Oxidative Stress on Male Fertility

Oxidative stress can have numerous effects on male fertility. One of the most significant effects is on sperm DNA. ROS can cause damage to sperm DNA, leading to genetic abnormalities that can affect fertility [50]. In addition, ROS can damage the sperm cell membrane, leading to decreased motility and viability. Oxidative stress can also lead to an increase in white blood cells in semen, which can further contribute to oxidative stress [44]. Finally, oxidative stress has been linked to a decrease in testosterone levels, which can affect fertility [28].

Lipid Peroxidation and Male Infertility

Lipid peroxidation is a natural process that takes place in the body when oxygen and free radicals react with the polyunsaturated fatty acids that are present in the cell membrane. This results in the formation of peroxides and aldehydes, which can be toxic to the cells. However, under normal circumstances, the body has a system of antioxidants that neutralize these toxic substances and prevent damage to the cell membrane [53]. The process of lipid peroxidation can occur due to various reasons, such as exposure to environmental toxins, stress, and an unhealthy diet. In recent years, researchers have begun to explore the link between lipid peroxidation and male infertility. Male infertility is a condition in which a man is unable to impregnate a woman due to factors such as low sperm count, poor sperm motility, and abnormal sperm morphology. This condition affects around 7% of men worldwide and is a major cause of infertility in couples. In this chapter, we will explore the relationship between lipid peroxidation and male infertility and the mechanisms involved. Sperm cells are particularly vulnerable to damage from lipid peroxidation due to their high concentration of polyunsaturated fatty acids. These fatty acids are essential for the proper functioning of the sperm cell membrane, which is crucial for maintaining the integrity and function of the sperm cell. Studies have shown that the level of lipid peroxidation is significantly higher in infertile men compared to fertile men [54]. This suggests that oxidative stress due to lipid peroxidation is a potential cause of male infertility. Lipid peroxidation can cause damage to the sperm cell membrane, which can result in a reduction in sperm motility, viability, and function. The production of reactive oxygen species (ROS) due to lipid peroxidation can also cause DNA damage, which can lead to abnormalities in sperm morphology. Furthermore, lipid peroxidation can affect the energy metabolism of the sperm cell by disrupting the activity of the mitochondrial electron transport chain. This can result in a reduction in ATP production, which is essential for sperm motility and function [53, 54].

Impact of oxidative stress and sperm DNA fragmentation on male fertility:
Sperm DNA fragmentation (SDF) stands as a pivotal factor in male infertility.
SDF signifies breaks in the DNA strands or alterations in nucleotide sequences.
Various factors like oxidative stress, chemical exposure, infection, and aging can
instigate SDF, thus presenting obstacles to male reproductive health [50]. The
impact of SDF on male fertility ranges from mild to severe. It is implicated in
reducing sperm motility, lowering fertilization rates, impeding embryo
development, and escalating miscarriage rates. Substantial research has linked
SDF with male infertility, and it is becoming increasingly apparent that high
levels of SDF can drastically impact reproductive outcomes. Crucial for male
fertility, sperm quality is negatively impacted by SDF. This can result in
diminished sperm concentration, poor motility, and abnormal morphology.
Moreover, sperm with high levels of SDF may have compromised DNA integrity,
leading to decreased fertilization rates and impaired embryo development [55].
Fertilization can also be detrimentally affected by SDF. Elevated levels of SDF
can decrease fertilization rates, thereby impeding conception. Studies have
indicated that men with high SDF levels have significantly reduced chances of
achieving pregnancy compared to those with normal SDF levels [56].

Embryo development, pivotal in the success of assisted reproductive technology
(ART), can be hindered by high SDF levels. This results in diminished embryo
quality and decreased pregnancy rates. Embryos derived from sperm with
elevated SDF levels have been associated with lower implantation rates and an
increased risk of miscarriage. For couples attempting to conceive, miscarriage is a
devastating outcome. High levels of SDF can increase this risk. Research
indicates that men with high SDF levels are more likely to have partners who
experience recurrent miscarriages than men with normal SDF levels [56]. Thus,
SDF poses a significant risk to male fertility, affecting several aspects, from
sperm quality to fertilization rates and embryo development, ultimately increasing
the risk of miscarriage. Future research and interventions should focus on
understanding and mitigating the factors causing high SDF levels.

Oxidative stress, apoptosis, and male infertility: The male reproductive system
is highly dependent on the proper functioning of germ cells, which are responsible
for the production of sperm. These cells are highly sensitive to oxidative stress
due to the high levels of ROS produced during spermatogenesis. Additionally,
sperm cells are highly susceptible to apoptosis due to the presence of numerous
checkpoints throughout their development that ensure their proper maturation.
When these processes are disrupted, it can lead to male infertility. Oxidative stress
can cause damage to sperm DNA, proteins, and lipids, which can impair their
function and reduce their fertilization potential [50]. ROS can also impair the
function of the mitochondria, which are essential for energy production in sperm

cells. This can lead to a decrease in motility and vitality, which are key factors for successful fertilization. Moreover, ROS can activate apoptotic pathways, leading to the death of sperm cells. Apoptosis is a highly regulated process that is essential for maintaining the quality and quantity of sperm cells. It occurs at various stages of spermatogenesis and is critical for the elimination of abnormal or damaged cells. However, excessive or inappropriate activation of apoptotic pathways can lead to a decrease in the number of viable sperm cells, which can result in male infertility. Studies have shown that oxidative stress can trigger apoptosis in germ cells, which can further exacerbate the detrimental effects of ROS on male fertility [57 - 59].

Several mechanisms have been proposed to explain the link between oxidative stress, apoptosis, and male infertility [57]. One of the main pathways is the activation of the nuclear factor kappa B (NF-κB) pathway, which is a key regulator of inflammation and cell survival. Under normal conditions, NF-κB is sequestered in the cytoplasm by the inhibitor of kappa B (IκB) proteins. However, oxidative stress can activate the IκB kinase (IKK) complex, which phosphorylates IκB and leads to its degradation. This releases NF-κB, which translocates to the nucleus and activates the transcription of pro-inflammatory and pro-apoptotic genes. This can lead to the activation of apoptotic pathways and the death of germ cells. Another mechanism is the activation of the c-Jun N-terminal kinase (JNK) pathway. JNK is a member of the mitogen-activated protein kinase (MAPK) family and is activated in response to various stress signals, including oxidative stress. JNK can phosphorylate and activate several transcription factors, including c-Jun, which can induce the expression of pro-apoptotic genes. Additionally, JNK can directly phosphorylate and inactivate anti-apoptotic proteins, such as Bcl-2, which can further promote apoptosis [60].

Antioxidants in the Treatment of Male Infertility

Antioxidants are compounds that can prevent or slow down oxidative damage in cells. They work by neutralizing free radicals, which are highly reactive molecules that can damage cells and cause aging, inflammation, and disease. Antioxidants are present in many foods and supplements, and they are known to have many health benefits, including reducing the risk of cancer, heart disease, and diabetes [61]. However, recent studies have also suggested that antioxidants may have a positive impact on male fertility. Male infertility is a common problem that affects around 7% of men in the US. It can be caused by a variety of factors, including hormonal imbalances, genetic disorders, infections, and lifestyle factors such as smoking, alcohol consumption, and poor diet. Oxidative stress is also a known factor that can contribute to male infertility. When there is an imbalance between free radicals and antioxidants in the body, it can cause oxidative damage to sperm and reduce their quality and motility [62]. Studies have shown that antioxidants can help reduce oxidative stress and improve sperm quality. For example, one study found that men who took a daily supplement of vitamin E and selenium for three months had significantly higher sperm motility and lower levels of DNA damage compared to a control group. Another study found that men who took a combination of antioxidants, including vitamin C, vitamin E, and CoQ10, had higher levels of sperm count, motility, and morphology compared to a placebo group. One of the reasons why antioxidants may have a positive impact on male fertility is that they can protect sperm from oxidative damage. Sperm are highly susceptible to oxidative stress because they contain high levels of polyunsaturated fatty acids, which are easily oxidized by free radicals. Antioxidants can help to neutralize free radicals and protect the sperm from oxidative damage, which can improve their quality and motility. Another way that antioxidants may improve male fertility is by reducing inflammation. Inflammation is a common factor that can contribute to male infertility, and it is often associated with oxidative stress. Antioxidants can help to reduce inflammation by neutralizing free radicals and inhibiting the production of inflammatory cytokines. This can improve the overall health of the reproductive system and increase the chances of successful conception [63].

However, it is important to note that not all antioxidants are created equal, and some may be more effective than others at improving male fertility. For example, vitamin C and vitamin E are both known to have antioxidant properties, but they have different mechanisms of action and may have different effects on sperm quality [61]. It is also important to consider the dosage and duration of antioxidant supplementation, as excessive intake of some antioxidants may have negative effects on fertility. In conclusion, antioxidants may have a positive impact on male fertility by reducing oxidative stress, protecting sperm from oxidative damage, and reducing inflammation. However, more research is needed to determine the optimal dosage and duration of antioxidant supplementation, as well as the most effective combination of antioxidants for improving male fertility. Men who are experiencing infertility should consult with a healthcare professional to determine the underlying cause and the best treatment options [63].

FUTURE DIRECTIONS IN RESEARCH

Despite the progress made in our understanding of the molecular mechanisms underlying male infertility, several critical research areas require further exploration to pave the way for more effective diagnostics and therapeutics.

Genomic and Epigenomic Studies

With the advent of next-generation sequencing technologies, more comprehensive genomic and epigenomic studies should be pursued to uncover novel genetic variants and epigenetic modifications associated with male infertility. Greater emphasis should be placed on non-coding RNA elements and their role in spermatogenesis and sperm function [8].

Single-Cell Genomics

A deeper understanding of the heterogeneity within the testicular cell population is needed. Single-cell genomics holds great potential in elucidating the complex interactions between different cell types in the testis, including germ cells, Sertoli cells, and Leydig cells [8].

Functional Validation of Genetic Variants

While genetic studies might identify potential disease-causing variants, functional validation in relevant models is needed to confirm their pathogenicity. Future work should focus on developing efficient *in vitro* and *in vivo* models to study the effects of these genetic variations on sperm production and function [64].

Environmental and Lifestyle Factors

Considering the influence of environmental and lifestyle factors on male fertility, comprehensive epidemiological studies need to be performed. These studies can provide insights into the interplay between genetic susceptibility and environmental exposures, which can be critical for devising preventative strategies [14, 65].

Advanced Assisted Reproductive Technologies (ARTs)

As our understanding of sperm biology improves, there will be new opportunities to enhance existing ARTs. For instance, sperm selection methods can be refined to identify the most viable sperm for use in procedures like intracytoplasmic sperm injection (ICSI) [56, 66].

Personalized Medicine

The ultimate goal is to transition from a one-size-fits-all approach to personalized treatment strategies for male infertility. The development of predictive models integrating genetic, epigenetic, and environmental risk factors will be key to achieving this goal. The future of male infertility research holds significant promise. Advancements in genomics, reproductive biology, and bioinformatics will be instrumental in unraveling the intricate mechanisms of male infertility, opening new doors for diagnosis and treatment [67].

CONCLUSION

The process of sperm maturation, including spermatogenesis, pre-capacitation, and capacitation stages, is crucial for successful fertilization. Any disruptions in these processes can result in male infertility. Factors such as gene mutations, abnormal sperm motility, hormonal imbalances, and oxidative stress contribute significantly to male infertility. Understanding these causes can help in the design of effective therapeutic strategies.

Male infertility at the molecular level is complex and multifactorial. Gene mutations may affect normal sperm development and function, while hormonal imbalances can disrupt the endocrine regulation of spermatogenesis. Oxidative stress can cause sperm DNA damage and reduce sperm quality and function. Genomic and epigenomic studies, single-cell genomics, and functional validation of genetic variants offer new opportunities to understand the molecular underpinnings of male infertility. Further research is also needed to understand how environmental and lifestyle factors affect sperm development and function.

The development and optimization of ARTs have a significant role in managing male infertility, providing potential treatment options for those affected. Given the varied causes and mechanisms of male infertility, personalized medicine approaches, which consider the unique genetic, hormonal, and environmental factors of each individual, may hold promise for improved diagnosis and treatment.

Male infertility is a complex condition with numerous potential causes, each with its distinct molecular mechanisms. Advancements in genomic technologies and personalized medicine, as well as a further understanding of the biology of sperm development and function, will be crucial in improving diagnosis and treatment strategies for male infertility.

REFERENCES

[1]   Agarwal A, Mulgund A, Hamada A, Chyatte MR. A unique view on male infertility around the globe. Reprod Biol Endocrinol 2015; 13(1): 37.
[http://dx.doi.org/10.1186/s12958-015-0032-1] [PMID: 25928197]

[2]   Olayemi F. Review on some causes of male infertility. Afr J Biotechnol 2010; 9.

[3]   Sengupta P, Dutta S, Krajewska-Kulak E. The disappearing sperms: analysis of reports published between 1980 and 2015. Am J Men Health 2017; 11(4): 1279-304.
[http://dx.doi.org/10.1177/1557988316643383] [PMID: 27099345]

[4]   Plante M, de Lamirande E, Gagnon C. Reactive oxygen species released by activated neutrophils, but not by deficient spermatozoa, are sufficient to affect normal sperm motility. Fertil Steril 1994; 62(2):

387-93.
[http://dx.doi.org/10.1016/S0015-0282(16)56895-2] [PMID: 8034089]

[5]   Wiersema NJ, Drukker AJ, Dung MBT, Nhu GH, Nhu NT, Lambalk CB. Consequences of infertility in developing countries: results of a questionnaire and interview survey in the South of Vietnam. J Transl Med 2006; 4(1): 54.
[http://dx.doi.org/10.1186/1479-5876-4-54] [PMID: 17192178]

[6]   Kedem P, Mikulincer M, Nathanson YE, Bartoov B. Psychological aspects of male infertility. Br J Med Psychol 1990; 63(1): 73-80.
[http://dx.doi.org/10.1111/j.2044-8341.1990.tb02858.x] [PMID: 2331455]

[7]   Leung AK, Henry MA, Mehta A. Gaps in male infertility health services research. Transl Androl Urol 2018; 7(S3) (Suppl. 3): S303-9.
[http://dx.doi.org/10.21037/tau.2018.05.03] [PMID: 30159236]

[8]   Kovac JR, Pastuszak AW, Lamb DJ. The use of genomics, proteomics, and metabolomics in identifying biomarkers of male infertility. Fertil Steril 2013; 99(4): 998-1007.
[http://dx.doi.org/10.1016/j.fertnstert.2013.01.111] [PMID: 23415969]

[9]   Jodar M, Soler-Ventura A, Oliva R. Semen proteomics and male infertility. J Proteomics 2017; 162: 125-34.
[http://dx.doi.org/10.1016/j.jprot.2016.08.018] [PMID: 27576136]

[10]   Krausz C, Riera-Escamilla A. Genetics of male infertility. Nat Rev Urol 2018; 15(6): 369-84.
[http://dx.doi.org/10.1038/s41585-018-0003-3] [PMID: 29622783]

[11]   Okada H, Fujioka H, Tatsumi N, *et al.* Klinefelter's syndrome in the male infertility clinic. Hum Reprod 1999; 14(4): 946-52.
[http://dx.doi.org/10.1093/humrep/14.4.946] [PMID: 10221225]

[12]   Darbandi M, Darbandi S, Agarwal A, *et al.* Reactive oxygen species-induced alterations in H19-Igf2 methylation patterns, seminal plasma metabolites, and semen quality. J Assist Reprod Genet 2019; 36(2): 241-53.
[http://dx.doi.org/10.1007/s10815-018-1350-y] [PMID: 30382470]

[13]   Sengupta P, Banerjee R. Environmental toxins. Hum Exp Toxicol 2014; 33(10): 1017-39.
[http://dx.doi.org/10.1177/0960327113515504] [PMID: 24347299]

[14]   Sengupta P. Environmental and occupational exposure of metals and their role in male reproductive functions. Drug Chem Toxicol 2013; 36(3): 353-68.
[http://dx.doi.org/10.3109/01480545.2012.710631] [PMID: 22947100]

[15]   Durairajanayagam D. Lifestyle causes of male infertility. Arab J Urol 2018; 16(1): 10-20.
[http://dx.doi.org/10.1016/j.aju.2017.12.004] [PMID: 29713532]

[16]   Cuppens H, Cassiman JJ. CFTR mutations and polymorphisms in male infertility. Int J Androl 2004; 27(5): 251-6.
[http://dx.doi.org/10.1111/j.1365-2605.2004.00485.x] [PMID: 15379964]

[17]   Sha Y, Zheng L, Ji Z, *et al.* A novel TEX11 mutation induces azoospermia: a case report of infertile brothers and literature review. BMC Med Genet 2018; 19(1): 63.
[http://dx.doi.org/10.1186/s12881-018-0570-4] [PMID: 29661171]

[18]   Ferlin A, Arredi B, Foresta C. Genetic causes of male infertility. Reprod Toxicol 2006; 22(2): 133-41.
[http://dx.doi.org/10.1016/j.reprotox.2006.04.016] [PMID: 16806807]

[19]   Zarkower D. DMRT genes in vertebrate gametogenesis. Curr Top Dev Biol 2013; 102: 327-56.
[http://dx.doi.org/10.1016/B978-0-12-416024-8.00012-X] [PMID: 23287039]

[20]   Zarkower D, Murphy MW. DMRT1: an ancient sexual regulator required for human gonadogenesis. Sex Dev 2022; 16(2-3): 112-25.
[http://dx.doi.org/10.1159/000518272] [PMID: 34515237]

[21]   Ellnati E, Fossard C, Okutman O, *et al.* A new mutation identified in SPATA16 in two globozoospermic patients. J Assist Reprod Genet 2016; 33(6): 815-20.
[http://dx.doi.org/10.1007/s10815-016-0715-3] [PMID: 27086357]

[22]   Dam AHDM, Koscinski I, Kremer JAM, *et al.* Homozygous mutation in SPATA16 is associated with male infertility in human globozoospermia. Am J Hum Genet 2007; 81(4): 813-20.
[http://dx.doi.org/10.1086/521314] [PMID: 17847006]

[23]   Ben Khelifa M, Coutton C, Zouari R, *et al.* Mutations in DNAH1, which encodes an inner arm heavy chain dynein, lead to male infertility from multiple morphological abnormalities of the sperm flagella. Am J Hum Genet 2014; 94(1): 95-104.
[http://dx.doi.org/10.1016/j.ajhg.2013.11.017] [PMID: 24360805]

[24]   Yang X, Zhu D, Zhang H, *et al.* Associations between DNAH1 gene polymorphisms and male infertility. Medicine (Baltimore) 2018; 97(49): e13493.
[http://dx.doi.org/10.1097/MD.0000000000013493] [PMID: 30544445]

[25]   Xu K, Yang L, Zhang L, Qi H. Lack of AKAP3 disrupts integrity of the subcellular structure and proteome of mouse sperm and causes male sterility. Development 2020; 147(2): dev181057.
[http://dx.doi.org/10.1242/dev.181057] [PMID: 31969357]

[26]   Liu C, Shen Y, Tang S, *et al.* Homozygous variants in *AKAP3* induce asthenoteratozoospermia and male infertility. J Med Genet 2023; 60(2): 137-43.
[http://dx.doi.org/10.1136/jmedgenet-2021-108271] [PMID: 35228300]

[27]   Sengupta P, Arafa M, Elbardisi H. Hormonal regulation of spermatogenesis Molecular signaling in spermatogenesis and male infertility. CRC Press 2019; pp. 41-9.
[http://dx.doi.org/10.1201/9780429244216-5]

[28]   Nieschlag E, Behre HM, Nieschlag S. Testosterone: action, deficiency, substitution. Cambridge University Press 2012.
[http://dx.doi.org/10.1017/CBO9781139003353]

[29]   Röpke A, Tüttelmann F. MECHANISMS IN ENDOCRINOLOGY: Aberrations of the X chromosome as cause of male infertility. Eur J Endocrinol 2017; 177(5): R249-59.
[http://dx.doi.org/10.1530/EJE-17-0246] [PMID: 28611019]

[30]   Sunnotel O, Hiripi L, Lagan K, *et al.* Alterations in the steroid hormone receptor co-chaperone FKBPL are associated with male infertility: a case-control study. Reprod Biol Endocrinol 2010; 8(1): 22.
[http://dx.doi.org/10.1186/1477-7827-8-22] [PMID: 20210997]

[31]   Simoni M, Gromoll J, Höppner W, *et al.* Mutational analysis of the follicle-stimulating hormone (FSH) receptor in normal and infertile men: identification and characterization of two discrete FSH receptor isoforms. J Clin Endocrinol Metab 1999; 84(2): 751-5.
[PMID: 10022448]

[32]   Ferlin A, Vinanzi C, Garolla A, *et al.* Male infertility and androgen receptor gene mutations: clinical features and identification of seven novel mutations. Clin Endocrinol (Oxf) 2006; 65(5): 606-10.
[http://dx.doi.org/10.1111/j.1365-2265.2006.02635.x] [PMID: 17054461]

[33]   Bruysters M, Christin-Maitre S, Verhoef-Post M, *et al.* A new LH receptor splice mutation responsible for male hypogonadism with subnormal sperm production in the propositus, and infertility with regular cycles in an affected sister. Hum Reprod 2008; 23(8): 1917-23.
[http://dx.doi.org/10.1093/humrep/den180] [PMID: 18508780]

[34]   Gaffney EA, Gadêlha H, Smith DJ, Blake JR, Kirkman-Brown JC. Mammalian sperm motility: observation and theory. Annu Rev Fluid Mech 2011; 43(1): 501-28.
[http://dx.doi.org/10.1146/annurev-fluid-121108-145442]

[35]   Wallach E, Amelar RD, Dubin L, Schoenfeld C. Sperm Motility. Fertil Steril 1980; 34(3): 197-215.
[http://dx.doi.org/10.1016/S0015-0282(16)44949-6] [PMID: 6250914]

[36] Gunes S, Sengupta P, Henkel R, *et al.* Microtubular dysfunction and male infertility. World J Mens Health 2020; 38(1): 9-23.
[http://dx.doi.org/10.5534/wjmh.180066] [PMID: 30350487]

[37] Singh AP, Rajender S. CatSper channel, sperm function and male fertility. Reprod Biomed Online 2015; 30(1): 28-38.
[http://dx.doi.org/10.1016/j.rbmo.2014.09.014] [PMID: 25457194]

[38] Hildebrand MS, Avenarius MR, Fellous M, *et al.* Genetic male infertility and mutation of CATSPER ion channels. Eur J Hum Genet 2010; 18(11): 1178-84.
[http://dx.doi.org/10.1038/ejhg.2010.108] [PMID: 20648059]

[39] Ho K, Wolff CA, Suarez SS. CatSper-null mutant spermatozoa are unable to ascend beyond the oviductal reservoir. Reprod Fertil Dev 2009; 21(2): 345-50.
[http://dx.doi.org/10.1071/RD08183] [PMID: 19210926]

[40] Eddy EM, Toshimori K, O'Brien DA. Fibrous sheath of mammalian spermatozoa. Microsc Res Tech 2003; 61(1): 103-15.
[http://dx.doi.org/10.1002/jemt.10320] [PMID: 12672126]

[41] Turner RMO, Musse MP, Mandal A, *et al.* Molecular genetic analysis of two human sperm fibrous sheath proteins, AKAP4 and AKAP3, in men with dysplasia of the fibrous sheath. J Androl 2001; 22(2): 302-15.
[http://dx.doi.org/10.1002/j.1939-4640.2001.tb02184.x] [PMID: 11229805]

[42] Zhu F, Wang F, Yang X, *et al.* Biallelic SUN5 mutations cause autosomal-recessive acephalic spermatozoa syndrome. Am J Hum Genet 2016; 99(4): 942-9.
[http://dx.doi.org/10.1016/j.ajhg.2016.08.004] [PMID: 27640305]

[43] Bak CW, Seok HH, Song SH, Kim ES, Her YS, Yoon TK. Hormonal imbalances and psychological scars left behind in infertile men. J Androl 2012; 33(2): 181-9.
[http://dx.doi.org/10.2164/jandrol.110.012351] [PMID: 21546616]

[44] Dutta S, Sengupta P, Muhamad S. Male reproductive hormones and semen quality. Asian Pac J Reprod 2019; 8(5): 189-94.
[http://dx.doi.org/10.4103/2305-0500.268132]

[45] Hiort O, Holterhus PM. Androgen insensitivity and male infertility. Int J Androl 2003; 26(1): 16-20.
[http://dx.doi.org/10.1046/j.1365-2605.2003.00369.x] [PMID: 12534933]

[46] Vineeth VS, Malini SS. A journey on Y chromosomal genes and male infertility. Int J Hum Genet 2011; 11(4): 203-15.
[http://dx.doi.org/10.1080/09723757.2011.11886144]

[47] Harton GL, Tempest HG. Chromosomal disorders and male infertility. Asian J Androl 2012; 14(1): 32-9.
[http://dx.doi.org/10.1038/aja.2011.66] [PMID: 22120929]

[48] Agarwal A, Sengupta P. Oxidative stress and its association with male infertility. Male infertility: contemporary clinical approaches, andrology, ART and antioxidants. 2020:57-68.
[http://dx.doi.org/10.1007/978-3-030-32300-4_6]

[49] Agarwal A, Leisegang K, Sengupta P. Oxidative stress in pathologies of male reproductive disorders Pathology. Elsevier 2020; pp. 15-27.
[http://dx.doi.org/10.1016/B978-0-12-815972-9.00002-0]

[50] Panner Selvam MK, Sengupta P, Agarwal A. Sperm DNA fragmentation and male infertility. Genetics of Male Infertility: A Case-Based Guide for Clinicians. 2020:155-72.
[http://dx.doi.org/10.1007/978-3-030-37972-8_9]

[51] Agarwal A, Finelli R, Durairajanayagam D, *et al.* Comprehensive analysis of global research on human varicocele: a scientometric approach. World J Mens Health 2022; 40(4): 636-52.

[http://dx.doi.org/10.5534/wjmh.210202] [PMID: 35118839]

[52]   Sengupta P, Dutta S, Alahmar AT. Reproductive tract infection, inflammation and male infertility. Chem Biol Lett 2020; 7: 75-84.

[53]   Fraczek M, Szkutnik D, Sanocka D, Kurpisz M. [Peroxidation components of sperm lipid membranes in male infertility]. Ginekol Pol 2001; 72(2): 73-9. [PMID: 11387994]

[54]   Aitken RJ. Free radicals, lipid peroxidation and sperm function. Reprod Fertil Dev 1995; 7(4): 659-68. [http://dx.doi.org/10.1071/RD9950659] [PMID: 8711202]

[55]   Dutta S, Henkel R, Agarwal A. Comparative analysis of tests used to assess sperm chromatin integrity and DNA fragmentation. Andrologia 2021; 53(2): e13718. [http://dx.doi.org/10.1111/and.13718] [PMID: 32628294]

[56]   Tournaye H. Male factor infertility and ART. Asian J Androl 2012; 14(1): 103-8. [http://dx.doi.org/10.1038/aja.2011.65] [PMID: 22179511]

[57]   Agarwal A, Said TM. Oxidative stress, DNA damage and apoptosis in male infertility: a clinical approach. BJU Int 2005; 95(4): 503-7. [http://dx.doi.org/10.1111/j.1464-410X.2005.05328.x] [PMID: 15705068]

[58]   Dorostghoal M, Kazeminejad SR, Shahbazian N, Pourmehdi M, Jabbari A. Oxidative stress status and sperm DNA fragmentation in fertile and infertile men. Andrologia 2017; 49(10): e12762. [http://dx.doi.org/10.1111/and.12762] [PMID: 28124476]

[59]   El-Taieb MA, Ali MA, Nada EA. Oxidative stress and acrosomal morphology: A cause of infertility in patients with normal semen parameters. Middle East Fertil Soc J 2015; 20(2): 79-85. [http://dx.doi.org/10.1016/j.mefs.2014.05.003]

[60]   Asadi A, Ghahremani R, Abdolmaleki A, Rajaei F. Role of sperm apoptosis and oxidative stress in male infertility: A narrative review. Int J Reprod Biomed (Yazd) 2021; 19(6): 493-504. [http://dx.doi.org/10.18502/ijrm.v19i6.9371] [PMID: 34401644]

[61]   Izuka E, Menuba I, Sengupta P, Dutta S, Nwagha U. Antioxidants, anti-inflammatory drugs and antibiotics in the treatment of reproductive tract infections and their association with male infertility. Chem Biol Lett 2020; 7: 156-65.

[62]   Gupta S, Sekhon L, Kim Y, Agarwal A. The role of oxidative stress and antioxidants in assisted reproduction. Curr Womens Health Rev 2010; 6(3): 227-38. [http://dx.doi.org/10.2174/157340410792007046]

[63]   Agarwal A, Sekhon LH. The role of antioxidant therapy in the treatment of male infertility. Hum Fertil (Camb) 2010; 13(4): 217-25. [http://dx.doi.org/10.3109/14647273.2010.532279] [PMID: 21117931]

[64]   Ding X, Schimenti JC. Strategies to identify genetic variants causing infertility. Trends Mol Med 2021; 27(8): 792-806. [http://dx.doi.org/10.1016/j.molmed.2020.12.008] [PMID: 33431240]

[65]   Leisegang K, Dutta S. Do lifestyle practices impede male fertility? Andrologia 2021; 53(1): e13595. [http://dx.doi.org/10.1111/and.13595] [PMID: 32330362]

[66]   Daar AS, Merali Z. Infertility and social suffering: the case of ART in developing countries. Current practices and controversies in assisted reproduction. 2002;15:21.

[67]   Garrido N, Hervás I. Personalized medicine in infertile men. Urol Clin North Am 2020; 47(2): 245-55. [http://dx.doi.org/10.1016/j.ucl.2019.12.011] [PMID: 32272996]

CHAPTER 3

Immune Homeostasis in the Male Reproductive System

Abstract: Testicular immune imbalance plays a considerable role in the origin of unexplained male infertility. The protection of spermatogenic cells from systemic immune reactions is crucial for maintaining standard spermatozoa generation. Since early postnatal development, the immune system is attuned to the auto-components of the host, yet sperm maturation first occurs during puberty. The variation in timing leads to the identification of spermatogenic proteins as foreign or antigenic. The creation of antibodies targeting these antigens triggers autoimmune responses, which can negatively affect sperm movement, functionality, and reproductive capability. Therefore, it is imperative for the testes to create a specialized immunoprivileged microhabitat that safeguards the allogenic germ cells. Protection of the testicles is achieved through a synchronized effort that includes different cells within the testes and native immune cells. The defense mechanism for the testicles entails isolating cells that could provoke an immune response by employing the blood-testis barrier alongside a combination of hormonal, local cellular signaling, immune-dampening, and immune-regulating processes. These complex processes require a combined theoretical understanding to clarify the physiological background and address immunogenic infertility caused by a dysregulated immune response in the testes. This chapter aims to (a) explain testicular immune privilege components, (b) describe how testicular somatic and immune cells interact to maintain the immune environment, and (c) show how various mechanisms work together to preserve this immune privilege.

Keywords: Androgens, Autoimmunity, Blood-testis barrier, Cytokines, Epididymis, Immune privilege, Immune response, Immunoregulation, Immunosuppression, Leydig cells, Lymphocytes, Male genital diseases, Orchitis, Prostatitis, Reproductive immunology, Seminiferous tubules, Sertoli cells, Spermatogenesis, Sperm auto-antigens, Testicular immune privilege, Vas deferens.

INTRODUCTION

Worldwide, 48.5 million couples are grappling with infertility, with male factors solely contributing to 20-30% of these cases, thus raising global health alarms [1, 2]. A thorough investigation has revealed that between 2.5-12% of men worldwide are infertile, with Central/Eastern Europe and Africa witnessing the

Sulagna Dutta & Pallav Sengupta

highest incidences of this issue [1], reinforcing the global significance of male infertility.

The intricate relationship between testicular cells and immune cells within the testes elucidates the intricate origins of male infertility [2, 3]. The distinctive anatomy of the testes, alongside their functional immunological advantage, promotes the establishment of a specialized immune microenvironment within this organ [4]. This distinct environment fosters tolerance towards sperm-associated antigenic proteins, shielding these foreign-like sperms from systemic immunological onslaught [5]. In the heart of the testes, two primary cell groups - somatic cells and immune cells - play an instrumental role in maintaining immunological equilibrium [6]. It is of paramount importance to shield the sperm-producing cells from the overall systemic immune responses - in other words, thwarting these auto-antigens from eliciting autoimmune responses is critical for preserving fertility in men [3]. This characteristic immunological forbearance of the testes towards various transplants is termed 'immune privilege'. However, ensuring this privilege demands intricate levels of immune control. Pathological states, like inflammatory conditions, infections, or congenital abnormalities disrupting testicular immune homeostasis, may instigate autoimmunity and immune-mediated infertility [7].

In recent years, numerous mechanisms underlying testicular immune privilege have been unraveled, but we are still a considerable distance from comprehending these processes in their entirety and collating this dispersed knowledge [8, 9]. An all-inclusive conceptualization of the disparity between systemic and testicular immune tolerance, the local immunosuppressive actions within the testes, and the roles of somatic cells, immune cells, and immunomodulatory molecules is indispensable for revealing the intricacies of maintaining testicular immune privilege - a crucial aspect for ensuring male fertility. This chapter aims to clarify the components of immune privilege in the testes, explore the connections among immune and somatic cells in the creation and maintenance of the immune-tolerant testicular microenvironment, and integrate the various mechanisms that significantly contribute to maintaining the testicular immune privilege.

THE UNIQUE IMMUNITY OF THE TESTES

Immune tolerance is established in the testes during the stages of puberty, serving to compartmentalize antigens generated by germ cells during spermatogenesis by the implementation of the blood-testis barrier (BTB) and specialized immunological cells [4]. BTB establishes a physical divide between the adluminal side of the germinal epithelium and antigens that can trigger autoimmune responses. However, it does not include all autoantigens associated with germ cells [4]. The production of anti-inflammatory cytokines and various growth factors enables the BTB to adopt an immunosuppressive function. This is enhanced by the creation of a tolerogenic atmosphere by tolerogenic-dendritic cells, Sertoli cells, and regulatory T cells (Tregs), all of which together play a vital role in establishing the immunosuppressive environment necessary for sustaining immune tolerance in the testis [4, 10 - 12]. The control of autoimmune reactions in the testes is achieved through both local and widespread cellular responses involving both tissue-specific cells and cells of the immune system. This allows for the expression of autoantigens by germ cells, aiding the process of spermiogenesis [13, 14]. Such coordinated processes are fundamental in establishing immunological tolerance in the testis.

ANATOMY OF TESTES AND IMMUNE HOMEOSTASIS

The architecture of the testis safeguards two principal functions: spermatogenesis and steroidogenesis. The execution of these roles necessitates a meticulous structural and anatomical configuration of the testis. The foundation for testicular immune privilege, indeed, is laid out by the specific arrangement of cells within the testicular tissue [4]. The seminiferous tubules and the interstitial area represent two distinct sections of the testis, separated by the blood-testis barrier (BTB) [4, 12, 15]. This particular structuring is fundamental to establishing the immune privilege observed within the testis.

Anatomical Characteristics of Seminiferous Tubules and Intestinal Space

In terms of histology and functionality, the testis displays a partitioned structure wherein androgen production and spermatogenesis transpire in discrete regions. Testosterone, a type of androgen, is generated within Leydig cells located within the interstitial zone, a space dispersed amongst the tubules. Spermatogenesis, on the other hand, unfolds within the seminiferous tubules, often referred to as the germinal compartment [6, 11, 13]. The genuine septa act in human infants for the segmentation of testicular lobules, extending from the fibrous enclosure known as the tunica albuginea that encapsulates the testis [16]. In mature human testes, these lobules are less pronounced, and in rodents, they disappear completely [16]. The seminiferous tubules are tightly curled tubes that start and end at the rete testis, housing the area where sperm begins to form [9]. Surrounding each tube, myoid tissues provide support and help squeeze the tubes through muscle-like movements [17]. These squeezing movements help move sperm, which cannot move on their own, from the seminiferous tubules to the rete testis and then to the epididymis [17]. However, the cells around the tubes do not fully stop substances from moving across their boundaries. Instead, these cells, together with Sertoli cells, produce various substances like growth factors and cytokines and are part of the base layer of the seminiferous tubules [18, 19]. Sertoli cells play a crucial role in the architecture of the seminiferous epithelium, extending from the bottom to the interior of the tubules. They aid in the maturation of sperm cells by supplying essential nutrients and growth factors [13].

Within the testis, specifically in the gaps surrounding the seminiferous tubules, Leydig cells are found. These cells are responsible for producing testosterone*via*a process known as steroidogenesis. Additionally, this region is home to immune cells, including macrophages, lymphocytes, mast cells, and dendritic cells. Their role is to safeguard the testis against infections potentially entering the bloodstream [13] Fig. (**5**).

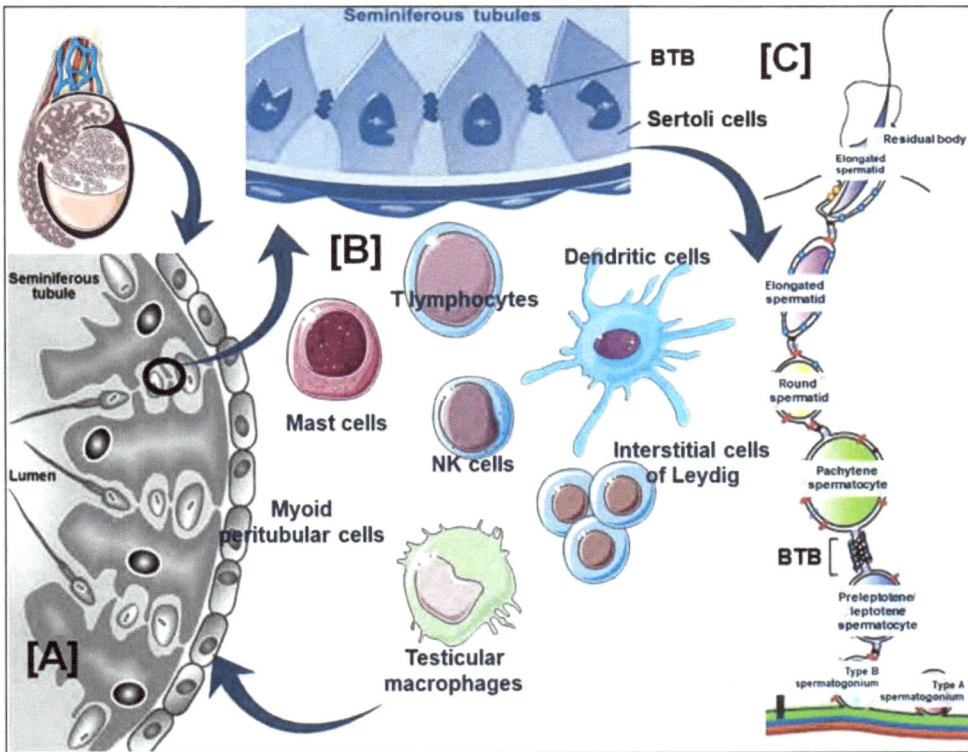

Fig. (5). Depiction of the unique anatomical and cellular elements that contribute to the immune-protective environment of the testes. (A) outlines the architecture of seminiferous tubules along with the areas surrounding them, referred to as interstitial compartments. (B) illustrates cells in the process of sperm formation in intimate association with supportive Sertoli cells; these cells are responsible for forming the blood-testis barrier (BTB) by means of tight junctions that prevent certain substances from crossing located near the bottom. (C) emphasizes the area within the testes known as the interstitial space, where Leydig cells responsible for synthesizing testosterone are located, as well as a variety of immune cells, including macrophages, dendritic cells, T cells, and mast cells, which are indigenous to this region.

Blood-Testis Barrier (BTB)

In the seminiferous tubules, the BTB forms through the intricate interactions between tight junctions, gap junctions, desmosome-like junctions, and basal ectoplasmic specializations among neighboring Sertoli cells. This structural integration plays a crucial role in isolating mature germ cells from the bloodstream.

The principal functionalities of the BTB are delineated within three synergistic domains: anatomical, physiological, and immunological, all of which collectively orchestrate the immunological milieu of the testes. The anatomical aspect of the BTB is characterized by the presence of junctional complexes that prevent mature (haploid) germ cells from entering the bloodstream [4]. On the other hand, the physiological dimension is underpinned by transport processes that are instrumental in crafting the interstitial milieu. Concurrently, the immunological facet is associated with the modulation of systemic immune responses and the suppression of autoantigenic germ cells' activity. However, upon the egress of spermatozoa from the seminiferous tubules, they are rendered susceptible to autoimmune assaults, attributed to the cessation of BTB functions at the rete testis [4, 20, 21].

The BTB was traditionally recognized for its role in maintaining the immunological sanctity of the testes by segregating antigens and antibodies until further findings revealed that spermatogonia and preleptotene spermatocytes could exhibit antigenic properties [4, 13]. The shift of preleptotene and leptotene spermatocytes from the basal to the adluminal compartment through the BTB is crucial for the conversion of diploid germ cells to haploid gametes. This shift ensures that post-mitotic germ cells, now outside the BTB's protective reach, do not trigger an immune reaction, thereby preserving the integrity of spermatogenic cells that develop after immune tolerance is established. This complex process requires the coordinated breakdown and rebuilding of junctional complexes among Sertoli cells as well as between the germ cells and Sertoli cells [11].

The regulation of BTB junctional dynamics is influenced by a constellation of cytokines, including interleukin 1-α (IL-1α), tumor necrosis factor-α (TNF-α), and transforming growth factor-β3 (TGF-β3), alongside other paracrine and endocrine signals [22 - 24], growth factors [25], and nitric oxide (NO) [26]. The organizational integrity of BTB is upheld by an assembly of adhesion proteins, notably through the synergistic actions of N-cadherin/β-catenin in gap junctions and occludin/ZO-1 in tight junctions, which are anchored to F-actin filaments, thereby furnishing the barrier with structural resilience [27]. Even though there has been a considerable restructuring of BTB to allow the movement of preleptotene spermatocytes, the immunological protection provided by the barrier is maintained throughout the cycle of the epithelium. This ensures that germ cells, both during and after meiosis, are safeguarded against immune system assaults [28]. The precise modulation of BTB dynamics is chiefly governed by the interplay of transforming growth factor (TGF)-β2 and testosterone, which orchestrate the opening and sealing of the BTB by selectively altering the trafficking of integral membrane proteins [29].

Nonetheless, the immune privilege of the testis cannot be ascribed to the BTB alone. The reconstitution of this specialized environment necessitates the synergistic interactions among various testicular somatic and immune cells, underpinning the complex regulatory mechanisms that ensure testicular immune privilege.

Testicular Interstitial Immune Cells

Research has elucidated the intricate organization of testicular interstitial tissue and its substantial lymphatic network, inclusive of continuous peritubular lymphatic sinusoids devoid of cellular connections with the seminiferous tubules or interstitium [30, 31]. These sinusoids encapsulate each seminiferous tubule and communicate*via*interstitial fenestrations, implying that any access to the seminiferous tubule necessitates lymph entry. Recent investigations indicate the location of lymphatic capillaries just beneath the tunica albuginea rather than within the interstitium. This was confirmed in an experimental rodent model where administered lymphocytes were observed migrating between seminiferous tubules and draining into the lymphatic vessels of the tunica albuginea [32]. Nevertheless, immune cells remain restricted from tubular access. The subsequent discussion will address the roles of various immune cells – macrophages, mast cells, dendritic cells, and lymphocytes– residing in the testicular interstitial space and their contributions to testicular immune homeostasis [32].

Macrophages

Macrophages are prevalent interstitial immune cells in the testis and are crucial for immunomodulation. They are divided into two main groups: anti-inflammatory ED2+ (CD163-expressing) macrophages, which upregulate IL-10 and secrete immunosuppressive factors, and pro-inflammatory ED1+ (CD68-expressing) macrophages, which secrete IFN-γ and TNF-α cytokines to induce inflammation [5, 33, 34]. A third subpopulation expressing both ED1 and ED2 is identified, which is unique for expressing nitric oxide synthase. For immune suppression in the testis, the ED2+ population dominates at 80%, leaving ED1+ at 20% [5, 33, 35 - 38].

Dendritic Cells

Dendritic cells, derived from bone marrow, are specialized antigen-presenting cells instrumental in lymphocyte activation and autoimmunity inhibition [13]. They optimize responses to foreign pathogens while minimizing autoantigen responses. In the normal testis, they express MHC class II, CD80, and CD86 similarly to during inflammation, but lower CCR7 mRNA and negligible IL-12p35 mRNA expression, indicative of an immature state, hence avoiding T cell activation and facilitating tolerogenesis [39 - 41].

Lymphocytes

Lymphocytes persist in the testicular interstitium under physiological conditions, largely comprising T cells, especially CD8+, and less CD4+, but no B cells. The population increases during inflammation or in infertility due to sperm autoimmunity, implying a role in adaptive immune responses [42, 43]. The testes contain immunoregulatory T cells, including CD4+CD25+ regulatory T cells and natural killer cells. Regulatory T cells inhibit antigen-specific immune response, playing a crucial role in immune tolerance. Studies on vasectomy models highlight their ability to balance tolerogenic and autoimmune responses to sperm antigens [6, 36]. Allograft experiments show memory T cell destruction and synthesis of graft antigen-specific regulatory T cells, suggesting their key role in testicular immune privilege, with potential significant roles of NK cells subject to future investigation [44 - 46].

Mast Cells

Mast cells play a critical role in testicular steroidogenesis, with elevated levels associated with male infertility [3, 4, 47, 48]. They stimulate collagen synthesis and fibroblast proliferation*via*the secretion of serine protease tryptase. Interestingly, mast cells affect regulatory T cells (Tregs) and immune tolerance [49 - 51]. While the exact mechanism remains elusive, it's known that mast cells can circumvent Treg-mediated suppression of effector T cells, necessitating T cell-derived IL-6 and the OX40/OX40L axis. In an experimental condition abundant in IL-6 and devoid of Th1/Th2 cytokines, activated mast cells can promote the transition of Tregs into IL–17–producing T cells, inducing inflammatory responses. Conversely, activated Tregs might recruit mast cells through IL-9, promoting regional immune suppression [52, 53].

Role of Testicular Cells in Immunity

The specialized cellular entities such as Sertoli Cells, myoid peritubular cells, and Leydig cells function as integral components in the sustenance of immunological equilibrium within the testicular milieu. Their role is underscored through a spectrum of immunomodulatory processes that are critical for maintaining this unique testicular immune privilege [13].

Leydig Cells

Leydig cells, predominantly found in the interstitial space, synthesize androgens, regulating spermiogenesis within the seminiferous tubules and influencing distal organs*via*peripheral circulation [54]. They exhibit immunosuppressive properties [55] by modulating the expression of pro- and anti-inflammatory cytokines in testicular cells and controlling testicular leukocyte count to limit excessive immune responses [56, 57].

Myoid Peritubular Cells

Myoid peritubular cells (MPCs), myofibroblast-like structures encircling seminiferous tubules, are instrumental in testicular development, spermatogenesis, and Sertoli cell functionality [58 - 60]. The MPCs-derived factor PModS is notable, which regulates the Sertoli cells' release of inhibin, transferrin, and androgen-binding protein [61, 62]. Additionally, mediators like heregulins, IGF-I, and other cytokines derived from MPCs mediate crucial interactions with Sertoli cells. MPCs, given their structural and locational characteristics, are posited to preserve testicular immune homeostasis. They contribute to testicular inflammation regulation by producing cytokines, leukemia inhibitory factor, MCP-1, TGPβ-2, and in humans, TNF-α receptors 1 and 2, recruiting inflammatory molecules, macrophages, and monocytes [63].

Sertoli Cells

Sertoli cells confer immunoprotection within the testis, facilitated by surface molecules and secreted factors. This property was demonstrated in a study involving co-transplanted allografts and xenografts in NOD diabetic mice, wherein the majority (64%) of recipients exhibiting Sertoli cell and islet grafts maintained normoglycemia 60 days post-transplantation, whereas solely islet-grafted mice did not. Immunochemical analysis disclosed elevated transforming growth factor (TGF)-β1 levels in Sertoli cell grafts of normoglycemic mice, implying a protective role against autoimmune attack, akin to normal testes defending developing germ cells [64].

Sertoli cells also aid phagocytosis, eliminating the residual bodies and germ cells undergoing apoptosis, which is integral for preserving testicular homeostasis [65]. This process aids spermatogenesis by ameliorating space constraints, averting harmful byproducts from necrotic, apoptotic germ cells, eliminating potential autoantigens, and recycling cellular components as an energy source. The process of phagocytosis by Sertoli cells is potentially facilitated through communication between class B scavenger receptor type I (SR-BI) and phosphatidylserine (PS) present on the surface of apoptotic cells. This mechanism is contingent upon the involvement of Tyro3, Axl, and Mer (collectively known as TAM) tyrosine kinase receptors in conjunction with their shared ligand, growth arrest-specific gene 6 (Gas6). Additionally, Sertoli cells play a pivotal role in modulating the immune response by suppressing the inflammatory activities of T lymphocytes and macrophages, thereby contributing to the immunological defense mechanism within the testicular environment [65, 66] Fig. (**6**).

Germ Cells

Spermatogonia, unlike later-stage germ cells, lack the blood-testis barrier (BTB) protection and are vulnerable to inflammatory insults. Despite this exposure, *in vitro* investigations reveal a subdued immune response to infection, possibly for testicular tolerogenicity maintenance [67]. Early spermatids and pachytene-stage spermatocytes also display a feeble immune reaction to viral challenges, albeit with minimal interferon (IFN) production [68]. Conversely, both meiotic and post-meiotic germ cells express Fas ligand (FasL), potentially regulating lymphocyte populations through apoptosis. Yet, germ cells alone insufficiently fend off viral threats. Sertoli and peritubular cells within seminiferous tubules, along with interstitial Leydig and immune cells, thus provide essential immunoprotection for germ cells, balancing immune responses to safeguard germ cell development [68 - 70].

INTER-CELLULAR NETWORKS IN TESTICULAR IMMUNE PRIVILEGE

Testicular immunity relies on robust intercellular networks involving germ cells, immune cells, and somatic cells) [6, 11, 12, 48]. Germ cells primarily interface with testicular macrophages (t-Mφ), dendritic cells, mast cells, regulatory T-cells (Tregs), natural killer T-cells (nk-TCs), and effectors T-cells. Within this framework, fully differentiated dendritic cells induce immunity dependent on T cells, whereas dendritic cells located within the testes promote a tolerogenic milieu, thereby safeguarding allogenic germ cells [39]. Similarly, t-Mφ, Tregs, nk-TCs, and MCs modulate testicular immunity, protecting germ cells from potential inflammatory responses [71].

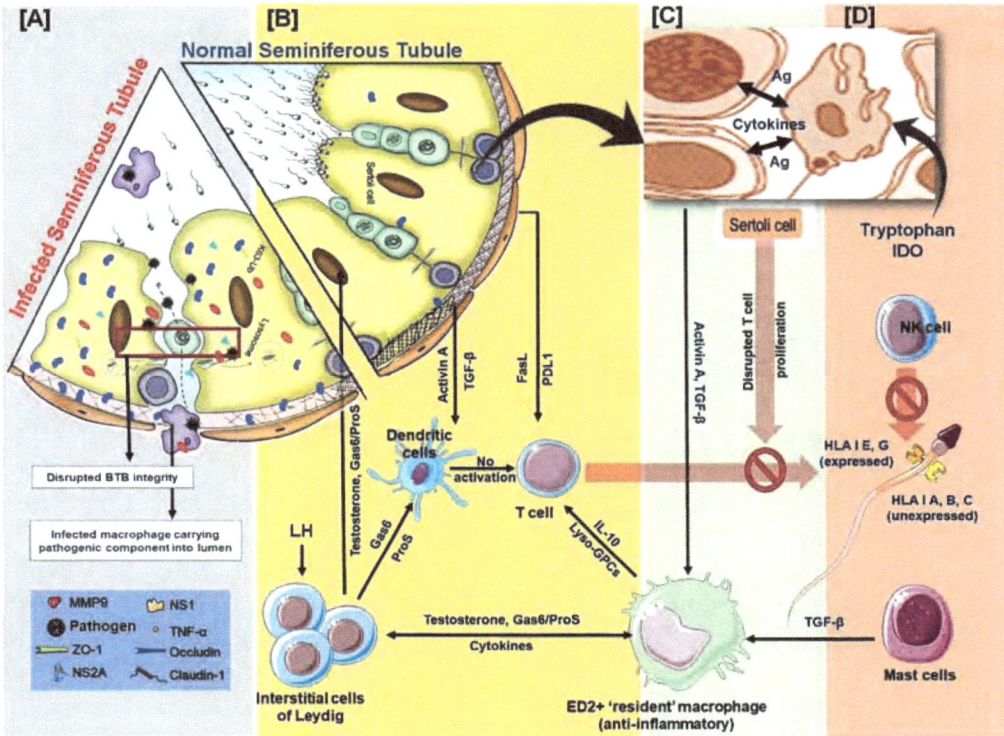

Fig. (6). The impact of testicular infections on testicular structure and function and the role of cellular communication and immune regulation in maintaining a protective environment for sperm development: (A) This figure illustrates how immune responses triggered by testicular infections can compromise the integrity of the blood-testes barrier (BTB) and damage the seminiferous tubules, negatively affecting sperm production across all stages; (B) In a healthy, infection-free seminiferous tubule, the BTB effectively isolates developing sperm cells (at various stages from pre-leptotene to mid-pachytene), including primary and secondary spermatocytes with self-antigens, from the surrounding interstitial area, safeguarding them against both local and systemic immune responses. Sertoli cells eliminate aging, apoptotic sperm cells, and excess sperm cytoplasm, thereby presenting sperm antigens to immune cells located within the testicular interstitium. This area is populated with immune cells such as macrophages, dendritic cells, T cells, and natural killer (NK) cells. Both Leydig and Sertoli cells regulate the population and functionality of testicular macrophages. Testosterone influences the activity of macrophages and dendritic cells to ensure that the presentation of sperm antigens leads to a tolerogenic (type 2) immune response, facilitated by the combined effort of regulatory factors from both somatic and immune cells, notably transforming growth factor β (TGFβ) and activin A from Sertoli cells, and the anti-inflammatory cytokine interleukin 10 (IL10) from macrophages and dendritic cells; (C) Concurrently, activated T cells are eliminated through mechanisms involving Fas ligand (FasL), indoleamine 2,3 dioxygenase (IDO), or lyso-glycerophosphatidylcholines (lyso-GPCs); (D) Furthermore, NK cells and CD8+ cytotoxic T cells are unable to identify sperm antigens due to the absence of classical HLA (Human Leukocyte Antigen) class I A, B, and C expressions. Consequently, specific adaptive immune responses against sperm antigens are either reduced or diverted, thus preserving sperm development and functionality. Interruptions in these processes can trigger autoimmune reactions against sperm antigens (a type 1 response), leading to uncontrolled inflammatory responses, the production of antibodies against sperm, the induction of germ cell death, impaired sperm function, and ultimately infertility.

Germ cells orchestrate apoptosis with the aid of immune cells, balancing viable and apoptotic environments. Testicular macrophages, for instance, regulate germ cell proliferation through inflammatory mediators like cytokines and nitric oxide (NO). This regulation involves the critical role of apoptosis markers like Bax, Bcl-xL, Fas, caspase 8, and soluble FasL, among others, in conjunction with cellular programming and testicular maturation [72, 73].

Interplay between Leydig cells and t-Mφ is integral to testicular functions, such as steroidogenesis and testosterone production. Inter-cytoplasmic digitizations facilitate this crosstalk by enabling intercellular transport of relevant factors. Leydig cell-stimulated macrophage proliferation and population maintenance also contribute to this interactive network [33, 34, 74 - 76].

Sertoli cells modulate macrophage, NK cell, and dendritic cell functions, establishing an immunosuppressive environment [3, 77]. They secrete factors like indoleamine 2,3 dioxygenase (IDO), transforming growth factors (TGF) β1−β3, activin A and B, and granzyme B inhibitors, which collectively serve to protect germ cells and suppress pro-inflammatory cytokines. Sertoli cells also express programmed death receptor-1/programmed death ligand-1 (PD-1/PD-L1), further inhibiting T-cell activation [6, 78 - 80]. Despite this understanding, the intricate mechanisms underpinning testicular immune homeostasis demand more comprehensive research.

FUNCTION OF ANDROGENS IN MAINTAINING IMMUNOLOGICAL EQUILIBRIUM WITHIN THE TESTES

Androgens, which are hormones like testosterone, have an important role in maintaining the testicular immune balance. They have been identified to mitigate inflammation and inhibit the immune response in this region [55]. These hormones work by directly affecting immune cells through specific receptors found on the cell surfaces, leading to changes in cell behavior, including how they move and secrete substances [81]. Research has consistently shown that androgens help protect the testicles from immune system attacks. For example, a study from 1985 discovered that blocking estrogen's effects in rats caused their bodies to quickly reject transplanted testicular tissue [82], with several other studies reporting similar outcomes [83 - 85]. It has also been found that androgens can control the number of certain immune cells within the testicles [57].

Recent studies further highlight androgens' protective role, especially in preventing inflammation in the testicles, such as in orchitis. They do this by reducing the production of inflammation-promoting substances and limiting the movement of immune cells like lymphocytes and macrophages into the testicles [9, 86]. Testosterone, one of the androgens, has been shown to increase a type of beneficial immune cell known as CD4+CD25+ regulatory T cells [12, 87]. A specific gene regulator, Foxp3, which is crucial for these beneficial immune cells to work properly, is influenced by androgens. This influence includes changes that help these cells function better [88]. In studies where rats had autoimmune orchitis, a condition where the body's immune system attacks the testicles, testosterone treatment was found to significantly increase these protective immune cells [86].

Despite these findings, the current research is not extensive enough to fully understand how androgens influence the immune functions of the testicles, highlighting the need for more detailed studies on this subject.

CONCISE MECHANISM AND SIGNIFICANCE OF IMMUNE HOMEOSTASIS FOR MALE FERTILITY

Immune homeostasis represents the orchestration of a fine equilibrium between the immune system's responsiveness to extraneous antigenic infiltrators and the body's inherent acceptance of its autologous tissues. This crucial balance becomes particularly significant within the male reproductive system, where its preservation is instrumental in safeguarding testicular tissue functionality, ensuring the optimal generation of spermatozoa, and maintaining the structural integrity of the male genital tract [89].

The testes exemplify an immunologically privileged locale that is biologically sequestered from the systemic milieu*via*the BTB [12, 29]. This complex arrangement of tight junctions segregates seminiferous tubules from interstitial tissues, operating as a selective filter to preclude immune cells and molecular entities, thereby creating a conducive environment for spermatogenesis. This characteristic is paramount as spermatozoa are haploid entities that express unique antigenic signatures, which, if exposed to the immune machinery, might trigger an immune response. Consequently, the conferred immune privilege permits unimpeded spermatozoan development devoid of potential immune-mediated rejection [90].

Despite the above isolation, immune cells can access the testes, although they are under rigorous regulation. The primary immune residents within the testes, the testicular dendritic cells, and macrophages, are pivotal in maintaining immune homeostasis. They uphold tolerance towards germ cells and bolster their maturation*via*growth factor secretion and phagocytosis of apoptotic cells. Additionally, they foster an anti-inflammatory milieu by secreting cytokines such as transforming growth factor-beta (TGF-β) and interleukin-10 (IL-10), which inhibit immune responses. Testicular macrophages embody unique phenotypic attributes and harbor functional specializations that augment spermatogenesis, distinguishing them from macrophages in other bodily regions [90].

Beyond the macrophages and dendritic cells, regulatory T cells (Tregs) significantly contribute to immune homeostasis within the testes. Tregs, a distinct subpopulation of T cells, facilitate immune tolerance by inhibiting the activation of other immune cells. Their presence within the testes is critical in averting autoimmune reactions against germ cells. Treg deficiency can precipitate autoimmune orchitis, a condition typified by testicular inflammation emanating from a self-directed immune attack against germ cells [91].

The epididymis, a highly specialized duct system that acts as a conduit connecting the testis to the vas deferens and facilitating sperm cell maturation and storage, is another focal point for immune homeostasis within the male reproductive system. The epididymis features unique immunological characteristics, shielded from immune cell incursion by tight junctions and the expression of immune regulatory molecules such as Fas Ligand (FasL), tumor necrosis factor-related apoptosis-inducing ligand (TRAIL), and nitric oxide (NO). Epididymal epithelial cells also secrete cytokines and chemokines that modulate immune cell recruitment and activation [92].

The prostate gland, an integral component of the male reproductive system, also contributes to immune homeostasis. The androgen-regulated prostate gland secretes seminal fluid, which is crucial for sperm motility and viability. The prostate gland manifests immunosuppressive molecules such as TGF-β and IL-10, promoting an anti-inflammatory environment. Furthermore, the prostate gland is a harbor for immune cells, such as macrophages and T cells, which uphold immune tolerance towards prostate-specific antigens and forestall autoimmunity [89].

Thus, immune homeostasis within the male reproductive system is of utmost importance for the preservation of fertility and overall reproductive health. The testes, epididymis, and prostate gland are immunologically privileged sites safeguarded from immune cell infiltration and sustain an anti-inflammatory environment. Immune cells.

CONCLUSION

The testis exhibits a unique environment, often described as immune-privileged, which protects developing germ cells from harmful autoimmune reactions. The unique anatomical structure of the testis plays a critical role in maintaining this immune homeostasis. Structures such as seminiferous tubules, the interstitial space, and the blood-testis barrier (BTB) serve as essential components of this system. The BTB, an important physical barrier between the bloodstream and germ cells, protects maturing sperm cells from being recognized as foreign by the immune system.

Immune cells, including macrophages, dendritic cells, lymphocytes, and mast cells, are present in the testicular interstitial space. They play roles in tissue maintenance, immune regulation, and response to infections. Tissue-specific cells such as Leydig cells, peritubular myoid cells, Sertoli cells, and germ cells contribute to local immune regulation within the testis, each playing unique and vital roles in maintaining testicular immune privilege. Complex intercellular networks within the testis contribute to immune privilege by fostering communication and coordination among different cell types. Androgens, primarily testosterone, significantly influence immune homeostasis in the testis. These hormones affect the functioning of various immune and testicular cells, thus modulating local immunity and inflammation.

Understanding the mechanisms of testicular immune homeostasis is crucial for male fertility, as imbalances can lead to conditions such as orchitis, infertility, and testicular cancer. Future research should focus on unraveling the intricate cellular interactions and molecular mechanisms underpinning testicular immune privilege. This understanding can contribute to the development of novel therapies for male fertility disorders and immune-related testicular diseases.

REFERENCES

[1]   Agarwal A, Mulgund A, Hamada A, Chyatte MR. A unique view on male infertility around the globe. Reprod Biol Endocrinol 2015; 13(1): 37.
[http://dx.doi.org/10.1186/s12958-015-0032-1] [PMID: 25928197]

[2]   World Health Organization Infecundity, infertility, and childlessness in developing countries. DHS Comparative Reports 2004; p. 9.

[3]   Zhao S, Zhu W, Xue S, Han D. Testicular defense systems: immune privilege and innate immunity. Cell Mol Immunol 2014; 11(5): 428-37.
[http://dx.doi.org/10.1038/cmi.2014.38] [PMID: 24954222]

[4]   Mital P, Hinton BT, Dufour JM. The blood-testis and blood-epididymis barriers are more than just their tight junctions. Biol Reprod 2011; 84(5): 851-8.
[http://dx.doi.org/10.1095/biolreprod.110.087452] [PMID: 21209417]

[5]   Meinhardt A, Wang M, Schulz C, Bhushan S. Microenvironmental signals govern the cellular identity of testicular macrophages. J Leukoc Biol 2018; 104(4): 757-66.
[http://dx.doi.org/10.1002/JLB.3MR0318-086RR] [PMID: 30265772]

[6]   Meinhardt A, Hedger MP. Immunological, paracrine and endocrine aspects of testicular immune privilege. Mol Cell Endocrinol 2011; 335(1): 60-8.
[http://dx.doi.org/10.1016/j.mce.2010.03.022] [PMID: 20363290]

[7]   Loveland KL, Klein B, Pueschl D, *et al.* Cytokines in male fertility and reproductive pathologies: immunoregulation and beyond. Front Endocrinol (Lausanne) 2017; 8: 307.
[http://dx.doi.org/10.3389/fendo.2017.00307] [PMID: 29250030]

[8]   Archana SS, Selvaraju S, Binsila BK, Arangasamy A, Krawetz SA. Immune regulatory molecules as modifiers of semen and fertility: A review. Mol Reprod Dev 2019; 86(11): 1485-504.

[http://dx.doi.org/10.1002/mrd.23263] [PMID: 31518041]

[9]   Fijak M, Bhushan S, Meinhardt A. The immune privilege of the testis Immune Infertility. Springer 2017; pp. 97-107.
[http://dx.doi.org/10.1007/978-3-319-40788-3_5]

[10]   Su L, Mruk DD, Cheng CY. Drug transporters, the blood-testis barrier, and spermatogenesis. J Endocrinol 2011; 208(3): 207-23.
[PMID: 21134990]

[11]   Smith BE, Braun RE. Germ cell migration across Sertoli cell tight junctions. Science 2012; 338(6108): 798-802.
[http://dx.doi.org/10.1126/science.1219969] [PMID: 22997133]

[12]   Fijak M, Bhushan S, Meinhardt A. Immunoprivileged sites: the testis. Methods Mol Biol 2010; 677: 459-70.
[http://dx.doi.org/10.1007/978-1-60761-869-0_29] [PMID: 20941627]

[13]   Li N, Wang T, Han D. Structural, cellular and molecular aspects of immune privilege in the testis. Front Immunol 2012; 3: 152.
[http://dx.doi.org/10.3389/fimmu.2012.00152] [PMID: 22701457]

[14]   Pérez CV, Theas MS, Jacobo PV, Jarazo-Dietrich S, Guazzone VA, Lustig L. Dual role of immune cells in the testis. Spermatogenesis 2013; 3(1): e23870.
[http://dx.doi.org/10.4161/spmg.23870] [PMID: 23687616]

[15]   Kaur G, Thompson LA, Dufour JM. Sertoli cells – Immunological sentinels of spermatogenesis. Semin Cell Dev Biol 2014; 30: 36-44.
[http://dx.doi.org/10.1016/j.semcdb.2014.02.011] [PMID: 24603046]

[16]   Liguori G, Ollandini G, Napoli R, Mazzon G, Petrovic M, Trombetta C. Anatomy of the Scrotum Scrotal pathology. Springer 2011; pp. 27-34.
[http://dx.doi.org/10.1007/174_2011_170]

[17]   Fleck D, Kenzler L, Mundt N, *et al.* ATP activation of peritubular cells drives testicular sperm transport. eLife 2021; 10: e62885.
[http://dx.doi.org/10.7554/eLife.62885] [PMID: 33502316]

[18]   Tripiciano A, Peluso C, Morena AR, *et al.* Cyclic expression of endothelin-converting enzyme-1 mediates the functional regulation of seminiferous tubule contraction. J Cell Biol 1999; 145(5): 1027-38.
[http://dx.doi.org/10.1083/jcb.145.5.1027] [PMID: 10352019]

[19]   Heinrich A, DeFalco T. Essential roles of interstitial cells in testicular development and function. Andrology 2020; 8(4): 903-14.
[http://dx.doi.org/10.1111/andr.12703] [PMID: 31444950]

[20]   Arck P, Solano ME, Walecki M, Meinhardt A. The immune privilege of testis and gravid uterus: Same difference? Mol Cell Endocrinol 2014; 382(1): 509-20.
[http://dx.doi.org/10.1016/j.mce.2013.09.022] [PMID: 24076096]

[21]   Doyle TJ, Kaur G, Putrevu SM, *et al.* Immunoprotective properties of primary Sertoli cells in mice: potential functional pathways that confer immune privilege. Biol Reprod 2012; 86(1): 1-14.
[http://dx.doi.org/10.1095/biolreprod.110.089425] [PMID: 21900683]

[22]   Sluka P, O'Donnell L, Bartles JR, Stanton PG. FSH regulates the formation of adherens junctions and ectoplasmic specialisations between rat Sertoli cells *in vitro* and *in vivo*. J Endocrinol 2006; 189(2): 381-95.
[http://dx.doi.org/10.1677/joe.1.06634] [PMID: 16648304]

[23]   Oduwole OO, Peltoketo H, Huhtaniemi IT. Role of follicle-stimulating hormone in spermatogenesis. Front Endocrinol (Lausanne) 2018; 9: 763.
[http://dx.doi.org/10.3389/fendo.2018.00763] [PMID: 30619093]

[24]   Syriou V, Papanikolaou D, Kozyraki A, Goulis DG. Cytokines and male infertility. Eur Cytokine Netw 2018; 29(3): 73-82.
[http://dx.doi.org/10.1684/ecn.2018.0412] [PMID: 30547889]

[25]   Catizone A, Ricci G, Caruso M, Ferranti F, Canipari R, Galdieri M. Hepatocyte growth factor (HGF) regulates blood–testis barrier (BTB) in adult rats. Mol Cell Endocrinol 2012; 348(1): 135-46.
[http://dx.doi.org/10.1016/j.mce.2011.07.050] [PMID: 21843593]

[26]   Lee NP, Cheng CY. Nitric oxide and cyclic nucleotides: their roles in junction dynamics and spermatogenesis Molecular Mechanisms in Spermatogenesis. Springer 2009; pp. 172-85.

[27]   Su L, Wang Z, Xie S, *et al.* Testin regulates the blood-testis barrier*via*disturbing occludin/ZO-1 association and actin organization. J Cell Physiol 2020; 235(9): 6127-38.
[http://dx.doi.org/10.1002/jcp.29541] [PMID: 31975378]

[28]   Mruk DD, Cheng CY. Sertoli-Sertoli and Sertoli-germ cell interactions and their significance in germ cell movement in the seminiferous epithelium during spermatogenesis. Endocr Rev 2004; 25(5): 747-806.
[http://dx.doi.org/10.1210/er.2003-0022] [PMID: 15466940]

[29]   Yan HHN, Mruk DD, Lee WM, Yan Cheng C. Blood-testis barrier dynamics are regulated by testosterone and cytokines *via* their differential effects on the kinetics of protein endocytosis and recycling in Sertoli cells. FASEB J 2008; 22(6): 1945-59.
[http://dx.doi.org/10.1096/fj.06-070342] [PMID: 18192323]

[30]   Clark RV. Three-dimensional organization of testicular interstitial tissue and lymphatic space in the rat. Anat Rec 1976; 184(2): 203-25.
[http://dx.doi.org/10.1002/ar.1091840207] [PMID: 942817]

[31]   Holstein AF, Orlandini GE, Möller R. Distribution and fine structure of the lymphatic system in the human testis. Cell Tissue Res 1979; 200(1): 15-27.
[http://dx.doi.org/10.1007/BF00236883] [PMID: 91443]

[32]   Hirai S, Naito M, Terayama H, *et al.* The origin of lymphatic capillaries in murine testes. J Androl 2012; 33(4): 745-51.
[http://dx.doi.org/10.2164/jandrol.111.015156] [PMID: 22052776]

[33]   Bhushan S, Meinhardt A. The macrophages in testis function. J Reprod Immunol 2017; 119: 107-12.
[http://dx.doi.org/10.1016/j.jri.2016.06.008] [PMID: 27422223]

[34]   Mossadegh-Keller N, Sieweke MH. Testicular macrophages: Guardians of fertility. Cell Immunol 2018; 330: 120-5.
[http://dx.doi.org/10.1016/j.cellimm.2018.03.009] [PMID: 29650243]

[35]   De Rose R, Fernandez CS, Hedger MP, Kent SJ, Winnall WR. Characterisation of macaque testicular leucocyte populations and T-lymphocyte immunity. J Reprod Immunol 2013; 100(2): 146-56.
[http://dx.doi.org/10.1016/j.jri.2013.09.003] [PMID: 24139314]

[36]   Wang M, Fijak M, Hossain H, *et al.* Characterization of the Micro-Environment of the Testis that Shapes the Phenotype and Function of Testicular Macrophages. J Immunol 2017; 198(11): 4327-40.
[http://dx.doi.org/10.4049/jimmunol.1700162] [PMID: 28461571]

[37]   Bhushan S, Tchatalbachev S, Lu Y, *et al.* Differential activation of inflammatory pathways in testicular macrophages provides a rationale for their subdued inflammatory capacity. J Immunol 2015; 194(11): 5455-64.
[http://dx.doi.org/10.4049/jimmunol.1401132] [PMID: 25917085]

[38]   Jarazo-Dietrich S, Jacobo P, Pérez CV, Guazzone VA, Lustig L, Theas MS. Up regulation of nitric oxide synthase–nitric oxide system in the testis of rats undergoing autoimmune orchitis. Immunobiology 2012; 217(8): 778-87.
[http://dx.doi.org/10.1016/j.imbio.2012.04.007] [PMID: 22672990]

[39] Rival C, Guazzone VA, von Wulffen W, *et al.* Expression of co-stimulatory molecules, chemokine receptors and proinflammatory cytokines in dendritic cells from normal and chronically inflamed rat testis. Mol Hum Reprod 2007; 13(12): 853-61.
[http://dx.doi.org/10.1093/molehr/gam067] [PMID: 17884838]

[40] Guazzone VA, Jacobo P, Theas MS, Lustig L. Cytokines and chemokines in testicular inflammation: A brief review. Microsc Res Tech 2009; 72(8): 620-8.
[http://dx.doi.org/10.1002/jemt.20704] [PMID: 19263422]

[41] Guazzone VA. Exploring the role of antigen presenting cells in male genital tract. Andrologia 2018; 50(11): e13120.
[http://dx.doi.org/10.1111/and.13120] [PMID: 30569647]

[42] Lustig L, Lourtau L, Perez R, Doncel GF. Phenotypic characterization of lymphocytic cell infiltrates into the testes of rats undergoing autoimmune orchitis. Int J Androl 1993; 16(4): 279-84.
[http://dx.doi.org/10.1111/j.1365-2605.1993.tb01192.x] [PMID: 8262661]

[43] El-Demiry MI, Hargreave TB, Busuttil A, Elton R, James K, Chisholm GD. Immunocompetent cells in human testis in health and disease. Fertil Steril 1987; 48(3): 470-9.
[http://dx.doi.org/10.1016/S0015-0282(16)59421-7] [PMID: 2957238]

[44] Samy ET, Parker LA, Sharp CP, Tung KSK. Continuous control of autoimmune disease by antigen-dependent polyclonal CD4+CD25+ regulatory T cells in the regional lymph node. J Exp Med 2005; 202(6): 771-81.
[http://dx.doi.org/10.1084/jem.20041033] [PMID: 16172257]

[45] Dai Z, Nasr IW, Reel M, *et al.* Impaired recall of CD8 memory T cells in immunologically privileged tissue. J Immunol 2005; 174(3): 1165-70.
[http://dx.doi.org/10.4049/jimmunol.174.3.1165] [PMID: 15661869]

[46] Nasr IW, Wang Y, Gao G, *et al.* Testicular immune privilege promotes transplantation tolerance by altering the balance between memory and regulatory T cells. J Immunol 2005; 174(10): 6161-8.
[http://dx.doi.org/10.4049/jimmunol.174.10.6161] [PMID: 15879112]

[47] Huang C, Wang Y, Li X, *et al.* Clinical features of patients infected with 2019 novel coronavirus in Wuhan, China. Lancet 2020; 395(10223): 497-506.
[http://dx.doi.org/10.1016/S0140-6736(20)30183-5] [PMID: 31986264]

[48] Chen Q, Deng T, Han D. Testicular immunoregulation and spermatogenesis. Semin Cell Dev Biol 2016; 59: 157-65.
[http://dx.doi.org/10.1016/j.semcdb.2016.01.019] [PMID: 26805443]

[49] Roaiah MMF, Khatab H, Mostafa T. Mast cells in testicular biopsies of azoospermic men. Andrologia 2007; 39(5): 185-9.
[http://dx.doi.org/10.1111/j.1439-0272.2007.00793.x] [PMID: 17714217]

[50] Yamanaka K, Fujisawa M, Tanaka H, Okada H, Arakawa S, Kamidono S. Significance of human testicular mast cells and their subtypes in male infertility. Hum Reprod 2000; 15(7): 1543-7.
[http://dx.doi.org/10.1093/humrep/15.7.1543] [PMID: 10875863]

[51] Frungieri MB, Weidinger S, Meineke V, Köhn FM, Mayerhofer A. Proliferative action of mast-cell tryptase is mediated by PAR2, COX2, prostaglandins, and PPARγ: Possible relevance to human fibrotic disorders. Proc Natl Acad Sci USA 2002; 99(23): 15072-7.
[http://dx.doi.org/10.1073/pnas.232422999] [PMID: 12397176]

[52] Eller K, Wolf D, Huber JM, *et al.* IL-9 production by regulatory T cells recruits mast cells that are essential for regulatory T cell-induced immune suppression. J Immunol 2011; 186(1): 83-91.
[http://dx.doi.org/10.4049/jimmunol.1001183] [PMID: 21115728]

[53] Lu LF, Lind EF, Gondek DC, *et al.* Mast cells are essential intermediaries in regulatory T-cell tolerance. Nature 2006; 442(7106): 997-1002.
[http://dx.doi.org/10.1038/nature05010] [PMID: 16921386]

[54] Rokade S, Madan T. Testicular expression of SP-A, SP-D and MBL-A is positively regulated by testosterone and modulated by lipopolysaccharide. Immunobiology 2016; 221(9): 975-85.
[http://dx.doi.org/10.1016/j.imbio.2016.05.005] [PMID: 27262512]

[55] Cutolo M, Sulli A, Capellino S, *et al.* Sex hormones influence on the immune system: basic and clinical aspects in autoimmunity. Lupus 2004; 13(9): 635-8.
[http://dx.doi.org/10.1191/0961203304lu1094oa] [PMID: 15485092]

[56] Wang J, Wreford NGM, Lan HY, Atkins R, Hedger MP. Leukocyte populations of the adult rat testis following removal of the Leydig cells by treatment with ethane dimethane sulfonate and subcutaneous testosterone implants. Biol Reprod 1994; 51(3): 551-61.
[http://dx.doi.org/10.1095/biolreprod51.3.551] [PMID: 7528551]

[57] Hedger MP, Meinhardt A. Local regulation of T cell numbers and lymphocyte-inhibiting activity in the interstitial tissue of the adult rat testis. J Reprod Immunol 2000; 48(2): 69-80.
[http://dx.doi.org/10.1016/S0165-0378(00)00071-1] [PMID: 11011073]

[58] Ailenberg M, Tung PS, Pelletier M, Fritz IB. Modulation of Sertoli cell functions in the two-chamber assembly by peritubular cells and extracellular matrix. Endocrinology 1988; 122(6): 2604-12.
[http://dx.doi.org/10.1210/endo-122-6-2604] [PMID: 3131119]

[59] Ramy RE, Verot A, Mazaud S, Odet F, Magre S, Le Magueresse-Battistoni B. Fibroblast growth factor (FGF) 2 and FGF9 mediate mesenchymal–epithelial interactions of peritubular and Sertoli cells in the rat testis. J Endocrinol 2005; 187(1): 135-47.
[http://dx.doi.org/10.1677/joe.1.06146] [PMID: 16214949]

[60] Mackay S, Smith RA. Effects of growth factors on testicular morphogenesis. Int Rev Cytol 2007; 260: 113-73.
[http://dx.doi.org/10.1016/S0074-7696(06)60003-X] [PMID: 17482905]

[61] Verhoeven G, Hoeben E, De Gendt K. Peritubular cell-Sertoli cell interactions: factors involved in PmodS activity. Andrologia 2000; 32(1): 42-5.
[PMID: 10702865]

[62] Maekawa M, Kamimura K, Nagano T. Peritubular myoid cells in the testis: their structure and function. Arch Histol Cytol 1996; 59(1): 1-13.
[http://dx.doi.org/10.1679/aohc.59.1] [PMID: 8727359]

[63] Schuppe H-C, Meinhardt A. Immune privilege and inflammation of the testis Immunology of Gametes and Embryo Implantation 88. Karger Publishers 2005; pp. 1-14.

[64] Suarez-Pinzon W, Korbutt GS, Power R, Hooton J, Rajotte RV, Rabinovitch A. Testicular sertoli cells protect islet beta-cells from autoimmune destruction in NOD mice by a transforming growth factor-beta1-dependent mechanism. Diabetes 2000; 49(11): 1810-8.
[http://dx.doi.org/10.2337/diabetes.49.11.1810] [PMID: 11078447]

[65] Nakanishi Y, Shiratsuchi A. Phagocytic removal of apoptotic spermatogenic cells by Sertoli cells: mechanisms and consequences. Biol Pharm Bull 2004; 27(1): 13-6.
[http://dx.doi.org/10.1248/bpb.27.13] [PMID: 14709891]

[66] Savill J, Fadok V. Corpse clearance defines the meaning of cell death. Nature 2000; 407(6805): 784-8.
[http://dx.doi.org/10.1038/35037722] [PMID: 11048729]

[67] Dejucq N, Lienard MO, Guillaume E, Dorval I, Jégou B. Expression of interferons-α and -γ in testicular interstitial tissue and spermatogonia of the rat. Endocrinology 1998; 139(7): 3081-7.
[http://dx.doi.org/10.1210/endo.139.7.6083] [PMID: 9645679]

[68] Dejucq N, Dugast I, Ruffault A, van der Meide PH, Jégou B. Interferon-alpha and -gamma expression in the rat testis. Endocrinology 1995; 136(11): 4925-31.
[http://dx.doi.org/10.1210/endo.136.11.7588226] [PMID: 7588226]

[69] Dejucq N, Jégou B. Viruses in the mammalian male genital tract and their effects on the reproductive

system. Microbiol Mol Biol Rev 2001; 65(2): 208-31.
[http://dx.doi.org/10.1128/MMBR.65.2.208-231.2001] [PMID: 11381100]

[70] Melaine N, Liénard MO, Guillaume E, Ruffault A, Dejucq-Rainsford N, Jégou B. Production of the antiviral proteins 2'5'oligoadenylate synthetase, PKR and Mx in interstitial cells and spermatogonia. J Reprod Immunol 2003; 59(1): 53-60.
[http://dx.doi.org/10.1016/S0165-0378(02)00061-X] [PMID: 12892903]

[71] Jacobo P, Guazzone V, Pérez C, Jarazo-Dietrich S, Theas M, Lustig L. Characterization of Foxp3+ regulatory T cells in experimental autoimmune orchitis. Transl Biomed 2010; 1: 72.

[72] Jacobo PV, Fass M, Pérez CV, Jarazo-Dietrich S, Lustig L, Theas MS. Involvement of soluble Fas Ligand in germ cell apoptosis in testis of rats undergoing autoimmune orchitis. Cytokine 2012; 60(2): 385-92.
[http://dx.doi.org/10.1016/j.cyto.2012.07.020] [PMID: 22892327]

[73] Lambrecht BN, Vanderkerken M, Hammad H. The emerging role of ADAM metalloproteinases in immunity. Nat Rev Immunol 2018; 18(12): 745-58.
[http://dx.doi.org/10.1038/s41577-018-0068-5] [PMID: 30242265]

[74] Winnall WR, Hedger MP. Phenotypic and functional heterogeneity of the testicular macrophage population: a new regulatory model. J Reprod Immunol 2013; 97(2): 147-58.
[http://dx.doi.org/10.1016/j.jri.2013.01.001] [PMID: 23415010]

[75] Svingen T, Koopman P. Building the mammalian testis: origins, differentiation, and assembly of the component cell populations. Genes Dev 2013; 27(22): 2409-26.
[http://dx.doi.org/10.1101/gad.228080.113] [PMID: 24240231]

[76] Giannessi F, Giambelluca MA, Scavuzzo MC, Ruffoli R. Ultrastructure of testicular macrophages in aging mice. J Morphol 2005; 263(1): 39-46.
[http://dx.doi.org/10.1002/jmor.10287] [PMID: 15536646]

[77] França LR, Hess RA, Dufour JM, Hofmann MC, Griswold MD. The Sertoli cell: one hundred fifty years of beauty and plasticity. Andrology 2016; 4(2): 189-212.
[http://dx.doi.org/10.1111/andr.12165] [PMID: 26846984]

[78] Sipione S, Simmen KC, Lord SJ, *et al.* Identification of a novel human granzyme B inhibitor secreted by cultured sertoli cells. J Immunol 2006; 177(8): 5051-8.
[http://dx.doi.org/10.4049/jimmunol.177.8.5051] [PMID: 17015688]

[79] Phillips DJ, de Kretser DM, Hedger MP. Activin and related proteins in inflammation: Not just interested bystanders. Cytokine Growth Factor Rev 2009; 20(2): 153-64.
[http://dx.doi.org/10.1016/j.cytogfr.2009.02.007] [PMID: 19261538]

[80] Cheng X, Dai H, Wan N, Moore Y, Vankayalapati R, Dai Z. Interaction of programmed death-1 and programmed death-1 ligand-1 contributes to testicular immune privilege. Transplantation 2009; 87(12): 1778-86.
[http://dx.doi.org/10.1097/TP.0b013e3181a75633] [PMID: 19543053]

[81] Sun YH, Gao X, Tang YJ, Xu CL, Wang LH. Androgens induce increases in intracellular calcium*via*a G protein-coupled receptor in LNCaP prostate cancer cells. J Androl 2006; 27(5): 671-8.
[http://dx.doi.org/10.2164/jandrol.106.000554] [PMID: 16728719]

[82] Head JR, Billingham R. Immune privilege in the testis. II. Evaluation of potential local factors. Transplantation 1985; 40(3): 269-74.
[http://dx.doi.org/10.1097/00007890-198509000-00010] [PMID: 3898493]

[83] Cameron DF, Whittington K, Schultz RE, Selawry HP. Successful islet/abdominal testis transplantation does not require Leydig cells. Transplantation 1990; 50(4): 649-53.
[http://dx.doi.org/10.1097/00007890-199010000-00024] [PMID: 2171164]

[84] Selawry H, Whittington K. Prolonged intratesticular islet allograft survival is not dependent on local steroidogenesis. Horm Metab Res 1988; 20(9): 562-5.

[http://dx.doi.org/10.1055/s-2007-1010885] [PMID: 3143654]

[85]   Whitmore WF, Gittes RF. Intratesticular grafts: the testis as an exceptional immunologically privileged site. Trans Am Assoc Genitourin Surg 1978; 70: 76-80.
[PMID: 753027]

[86]   Fijak M, Schneider E, Klug J, *et al.* Testosterone replacement effectively inhibits the development of experimental autoimmune orchitis in rats: evidence for a direct role of testosterone on regulatory T cell expansion. J Immunol 2011; 186(9): 5162-72.
[http://dx.doi.org/10.4049/jimmunol.1001958] [PMID: 21441459]

[87]   Walecki M, Eisel F, Klug J, *et al.* Androgen receptor modulates *Foxp3* expression in CD4 $^+$ CD25 $^+$ Foxp3 $^+$ regulatory T-cells. Mol Biol Cell 2015; 26(15): 2845-57.
[http://dx.doi.org/10.1091/mbc.E14-08-1323] [PMID: 26063731]

[88]   Hori S, Nomura T, Sakaguchi S. Control of regulatory T cell development by the transcription factor Foxp3. Science 2003; 299(5609): 1057-61.
[http://dx.doi.org/10.1126/science.1079490] [PMID: 12522256]

[89]   Wang F, Chen R, Han D. Innate immune defense in the male reproductive system and male fertility. Innate Immunity in Health and Disease 2019.

[90]   Dutta S, Sandhu N, Sengupta P, Alves MG, Henkel R, Agarwal A. Somatic-immune cells crosstalk in-the-making of testicular immune privilege. Reprod Sci 2022; 29(10): 2707-18.
[http://dx.doi.org/10.1007/s43032-021-00721-0] [PMID: 34580844]

[91]   Campese AF, Grazioli P, de Cesaris P, *et al.* Mouse Sertoli cells sustain *de novo* generation of regulatory T cells by triggering the notch pathway through soluble JAGGED1. Biol Reprod 2014; 90(3): 53.
[http://dx.doi.org/10.1095/biolreprod.113.113803] [PMID: 24478388]

[92]   Pelletier RM. The blood-testis barrier: the junctional permeability, the proteins and the lipids. Prog Histochem Cytochem 2011 Aug 1;46(2):49-127
[http://dx.doi.org/10.1016/j.proghi.2011.05.001] [PMID: 21705043]

CHAPTER 4

Immunological Factors of Male Infertility

Abstract: The intricate mechanisms underlying immunological causes of male infertility are progressively gaining prominence within the field of reproductive medicine. It is essential to articulate the functional significance of the unique nature of the testicular immune environment in the context of male reproduction. Additionally, considerable gaps persist in our comprehension of the detrimental impacts instigated by inflammatory cytokines on spermatozoa quality and motility. The present chapter explains the testicular immune components, immune tolerance and response, and also the etiological aspects of these immunological elements, emphasizing the potential role of genetic susceptibility, infection or trauma to the male reproductive tract, and environmental toxin exposure as contributory factors to male infertility. Moreover, this chapter provides an extensive review of the prevailing diagnostic methods, incorporating physical examinations, semen analysis, and anti-sperm antibody (ASA) detection procedures. The discussion is extended to the realm of therapeutic interventions, including the use of immunosuppressive regimens and assisted reproductive technologies (ARTs). This comprehensive chapter thus serves as a critical reference for grasping the intricate interaction between the immune system and male reproductive health, thereby facilitating the progression of efficacious fertility treatments and improvement in patient outcomes.

Keywords: Anti-sperm antibodies, Autoimmunity, Cytokines, Epididymis, Immunoglobulins, Immunological tests, Immunoreactive techniques, Infertility, Inflammation, Leydig cells, Orchitis, Reproductive immunology, Scrotum, Semen analysis, Seminal plasma proteins, Sertoli cells, Sperm agglutination, Sperm motility, Testis, Vas deferens.

INTRODUCTION

Infertility is a common problem that affects both men and women. According to the World Health Organization (WHO), approximately 15% of couples worldwide experience infertility. Out of these, male infertility is the sole cause in about 30% of cases, while in another 20-30% of cases, both partners have fertility problems [1].

The prevalence of male infertility varies depending on the population being studied and the criteria used to define infertility. In general, the prevalence of

Sulagna Dutta & Pallav Sengupta

male infertility has been increasing over the past few decades. It has been suggested that the prevalence of male infertility had increased from 8% in the 1980s to 12-14% in the 2000s [2].

The immune system plays a crucial role in male fertility by helping to protect the reproductive organs from infection and inflammation [3, 4]. One important aspect of the role of the immune system in male fertility is the presence of immune cells in the testes. The testes are normally considered immune-privileged sites, meaning that they are protected from the self-immune system to prevent damage to developing sperm cells. However, some immune cells are present in the testes to help control and maintain the immune balance in this sensitive area [5].

In addition, the immune system helps to protect the male reproductive system from invading pathogens that could damage or destroy sperm cells. The immune response may be triggered in response to infections or other insults, leading to inflammation and the recruitment of immune cells to the area to help clear the infection [6, 7]. However, an overactive immune response or chronic inflammation can also have negative effects on male fertility. In some cases, the immune system may mistakenly attack and damage healthy sperm cells, leading to infertility. Autoimmune disorders, where the immune system mistakenly targets its own tissues, can also affect male fertility [8, 9].

The present chapter explains how the immune system plays a complex and important role in male fertility, helping to protect the reproductive organs from infection and inflammation while also maintaining a delicate balance to avoid harming healthy sperm cells.

IMMUNOLOGICAL FACTORS IN MALE INFERTILITY

Male infertility is a complex condition that affects millions of men worldwide. While there are many causes of infertility, one important factor that has gained increasing attention in recent years is the role of the immune system.

Antisperm Antibodies (ASA)

Antisperm antibodies (ASA) are a type of immune response in which the body produces antibodies against sperm. These antibodies can bind to the surface of sperm cells, causing them to become immotile or agglutinate (stick together), which can impair their ability to fertilize an egg [10]. ASA can develop as a result of exposure to sperm outside of the reproductive tract, such as during a vasectomy, or as a result of damage to the blood-testis barrier, which normally protects developing sperm from the immune system. They can also develop as a result of an autoimmune condition, in which the body mistakenly attacks its own tissues. In men with ASA, the level and activity of these antibodies can vary widely, with some men showing no apparent effect on fertility while others experience severe impairment [10, 11]. ASA can be measured using a variety of tests, including the mixed antiglobulin reaction (MAR) test, the immunobead binding assay (IBBA), and the enzyme-linked immunosorbent assay (ELISA) [11].

Treatment for ASA-related infertility can include immunosuppressive therapy, such as corticosteroids, to reduce the level of antibodies. In some cases, assisted reproductive technologies, such as *in vitro* fertilization (IVF) or intrauterine insemination (IUI), may be necessary to achieve pregnancy [12, 13].

Role of T-cells and Natural Killer (NK) Cells

T-cells and NK cells are important components of the immune system that play a role in defending the body against infection and disease. In the context of male infertility, however, these cells can also contribute to damage to the testes and impaired sperm function [14].

T-cells are a type of white blood cell that helps to identify and eliminate foreign invaders, such as viruses or bacteria. In some cases, however, T-cells can become activated and attack the body's own tissues, including the testes. This can result in inflammation and damage to the testes, which can impair sperm production and quality [15]. NK cells are another type of immune cell that plays a role in defending against infection and cancer. In the context of male infertility, NK cells can also attack sperm cells, either by directly targeting them or by producing inflammatory cytokines that damage sperm function [14]. There is still much to be learned about the role of T-cells and NK cells in male infertility, and more research is needed to fully understand the mechanisms by which they contribute to the condition. However, some studies have suggested that reducing the activity of these cells, either through immunosuppressive therapy or other means, may be a potential avenue for improving fertility in men with immunological factors [14].

Inflammatory Cytokines and their Effects on Sperm Quality and Motility

The presence of inflammatory cytokines in the male reproductive tract can have a significant impact on sperm quality and motility. Cytokines are small proteins that are secreted by cells of the immune system. They act as messengers, communicating with other cells to coordinate the immune response to infection or injury. In the male reproductive tract, cytokines play an important role in maintaining a healthy environment for sperm development and transport. However, when the immune system becomes overactive, it can produce an excess of inflammatory cytokines that can damage sperm and impair fertility [16]. One of the most important cytokines involved in male infertility is tumor necrosis factor-alpha (TNF-α). This cytokine is produced by a variety of immune cells, including macrophages and T cells. In the male reproductive tract, TNF-α is produced by both the testis and the epididymis, where it plays a role in regulating sperm transport and maturation. However, when TNF-α levels become elevated due to infection or inflammation, it can have a negative impact on sperm quality and motility [17, 18].

Studies have shown that high levels of TNF-α in semen are associated with decreased sperm concentration, motility, and viability. TNF-α can also cause damage to the sperm cell membrane, leading to impaired function and increased susceptibility to OS [19]. In addition, TNF-α can interfere with the interaction between sperm and the female reproductive tract, making it more difficult for sperm to reach and fertilize the egg. Another important cytokine involved in male infertility is interleukin-6 (IL-6). This cytokine is produced by a variety of immune cells, including T cells, B cells, and macrophages. In the male reproductive tract, IL-6 is produced by the testis, epididymis, and seminal vesicles, where it plays a role in regulating sperm maturation and transport. However, like TNF-α, elevated levels of IL-6 can have a negative impact on sperm quality and motility [20].

Studies have shown that high levels of IL-6 in semen are associated with decreased sperm concentration, motility, and morphology. IL-6 can also cause damage to the sperm cell membrane, leading to impaired function and increased susceptibility to OS [21]. In addition, IL-6 can interfere with the interaction between sperm and the female reproductive tract, making it more difficult for sperm to reach and fertilize the egg. Other cytokines that have been implicated in male infertility include interferon-gamma (IFN-γ), interleukin-8 (IL-8), and interleukin-1 beta (IL-1β) [16]. IFN-γ is produced by T cells and natural killer cells and plays a role in regulating the immune response to infection. However, elevated levels of IFN-γ in semen have been associated with decreased sperm motility and viability [22]. IL-8 is produced by a variety of immune cells and plays a role in recruiting other immune cells to sites of infection or inflammation. Elevated levels of IL-8 in semen have been associated with decreased sperm motility and morphology [23, 24]. IL-1β is produced by macrophages and plays a role in regulating the immune response to infection. Elevated levels of IL-1β in semen have been associated with decreased sperm motility and viability [20].

CAUSES OF IMMUNOLOGICAL FACTORS IN MALE INFERTILITY

The immunological factors implicated in male infertility often include the production of ASAs, excessive pro-inflammatory cytokines, and alterations in the local immunosuppressive milieu within the male reproductive system. ASAs, for instance, can interfere with various stages of fertilization, from impeding sperm mobility and capacitation to blocking the acrosome reaction and sperm-oocyte fusion. This ultimately results in decreased sperm quality and fertility potential. In some instances, an aberrant immune response may occur due to the breakdown of the immune-privileged status of the testes, possibly resulting from infection, trauma, or surgical procedures. This leads to the recognition of sperm antigens by the immune system, thus eliciting an autoimmune response, which subsequently precipitates male infertility. Moreover, excessive pro-inflammatory cytokines and oxidative stress (OS) in the male genital tract may compromise the spermatozoa's ability to fertilize the oocyte effectively. These conditions can result in detrimental effects on sperm DNA integrity, causing DNA fragmentation and potentially leading to infertility, miscarriage, or developmental abnormalities in offspring [10].

One of the most common causes of immunological factors in male infertility is varicocele [25]. Varicocele is a condition where the veins in the scrotum become enlarged, leading to a buildup of blood that can negatively impact the temperature of the testes. This can lead to an increase in the production of antibodies against sperm cells. Studies have shown that men with varicocele are more likely to have higher levels of anti-sperm antibodies, which can lead to reduced sperm count and motility [25]. Another cause of immunological factors in male infertility is epididymitis, a type of inflammation that occurs in the epididymis. Approximately forty percent of the patient population experience persistent oligospermia or azoospermia, conditions that are intrinsically associated with the immunological features of the epididymis. Furthermore, the pathophysiological traits of epididymitis vary, contingent upon the specific pathogenic microorganisms inciting the infection [26, 27].

In some cases, the cause of immunological factors in male infertility is unknown. This is known as idiopathic infertility. In these cases, the immune system may be producing antibodies against sperm cells for no apparent reason. However, recent studies have shown that there may be a genetic component to idiopathic infertility, which may be responsible for the production of anti-sperm antibodies [28].

In addition to these causes, certain medical treatments can also contribute to immunological factors in male infertility. For example, men who undergo chemotherapy or radiation therapy for cancer may produce antibodies against sperm cells as a side effect of these treatments [29]. Similarly, men who undergo a vasectomy reversal may produce antibodies against sperm cells as a result of the surgical procedure [30].

Therefore, while the causes of immunological factors in male infertility vary widely, the resultant impact on fertility is generally similar - disruption of normal sperm function and a decline in reproductive potential. A comprehensive understanding of these immunological factors can pave the way for novel therapeutic strategies and diagnostics for male infertility.

Genetic Predisposition

In many cases, male infertility is caused by genetic factors that contribute to abnormal sperm production or function. Understanding the genetic basis of male infertility can provide insights into its diagnosis, treatment, and prevention [31]. One of the most well-known genetic causes of male infertility is Klinefelter syndrome. This is a chromosomal abnormality that occurs when a male has an extra X chromosome, resulting in a karyotype of 47,XXY. Men with Klinefelter syndrome often have small testes, reduced testosterone levels, and impaired sperm production. Another genetic cause of male infertility is Y chromosome microdeletions. The Y chromosome contains several genes that are essential for sperm production, and deletions in these regions can result in azoospermia (no sperm in semen) or oligospermia (low sperm count) Fig. (7).

In addition to the well-established genetic causes of male infertility, there is growing evidence of genetic alterations of the immunological milieu that contribute significantly to the pathogenesis of male infertility. Common polymorphisms in pro-inflammatory and anti-inflammatory cytokine genes may modify cytokine production and function in response to pathogens and could be a potential risk factor for male infertility [16, 32]. It is known that several cytokines, including interleukin 1, 2, 6, 18, TNFα, and soluble receptors of interleukin (SRIL) such as SRIL2 and 6, have a significant impact on sperm parameters and are involved in the process of spermatogenesis [33, 34]. The interleukin-1 family, comprising IL-1α, IL-1β, and IL-1RA, regulates the expression of proteins essential for proliferation, cell survival, and angiogenesis during spermatogenesis. Under typical testicular homeostasis, interleukin-1 is continuously expressed, fostering a unique microenvironment conducive to the conversion of diploid gametogenic cells into haploid spermatozoa, a process that intensifies during instances of inflammation and infection [35]. Disruption in the functions of cytokines and chemokines through their genetic polymorphism can precipitate male infertility by impairing spermatic functions. Various studies indicate a correlation between the single nucleotide polymorphisms, C3953T SNP in the IL-1β gene, and male infertility [36 - 38].

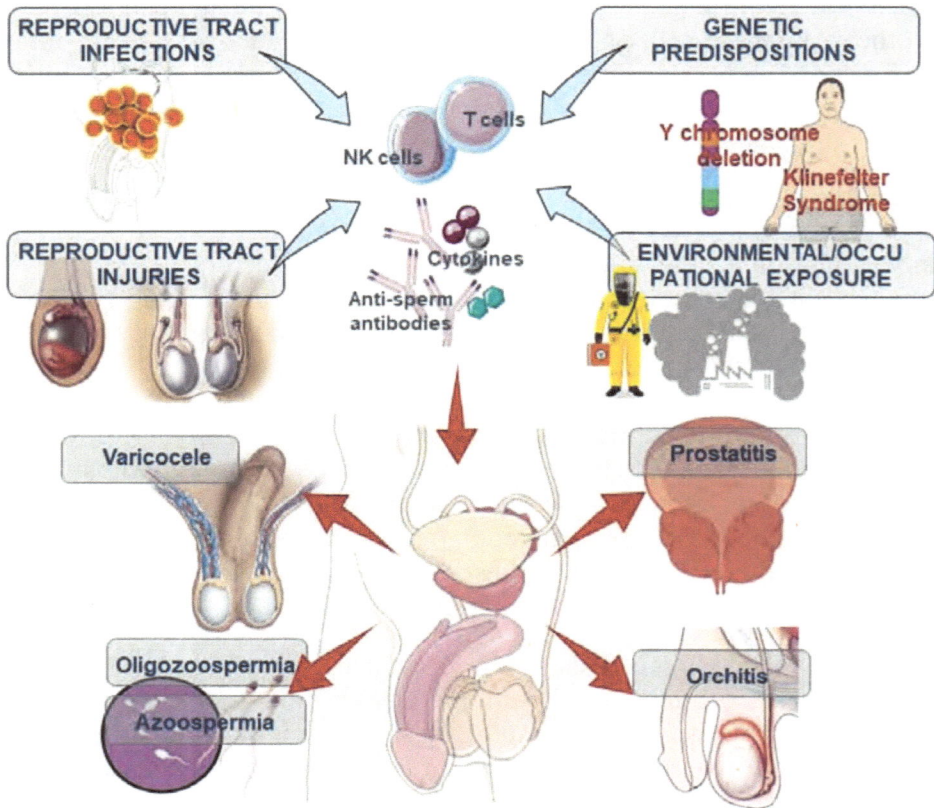

Fig. (7). Immunological factors of male infertility.

Genome-wide association studies (GWAS) have pinpointed multiple genetic variants related to sperm count, motility, and morphology, residing in genes pertinent to testicular development, hormonal regulation, and DNA repair, among others [39]. An interplay of these genetic and epigenetic variations with environmental and lifestyle variables may amplify infertility risks [40, 41]. One such environmental element is endocrine disruptors, ubiquitous in products like plastics, pesticides, and personal care items. These chemicals can disturb hormonal equilibrium and, over time, bioaccumulate. Exposure to endocrine disruptors like phthalates, bisphenol A, and organochlorines might impair male fertility*via*sperm count, motility, and quality reduction. Further, these chemicals could potentially modulate epigenetic markers on sperm DNA, influencing offspring health and development [40]. Obesity, a lifestyle factor, may also exacerbate the impacts of genetic susceptibility to male infertility [42, 43]. Hormonal imbalances associated with obesity, such as reduced testosterone and increased estrogen levels, can impair sperm production and function. Also, the pro-inflammatory state of obesity potentially escalates OS and sperm DNA damage, reinforcing obesity as a male infertility risk factor [43]. Notwithstanding the expanding comprehension of genetic and environmental contributors to male infertility, challenges persist in its diagnosis and treatment.

Infection or Injury to the Reproductive Tract

Infections and injuries to the male reproductive tract can affect the testicles, epididymis, vas deferens, prostate gland, and urethra. Infections can be caused by bacteria, viruses, and fungi [44], while injuries can be caused by trauma or surgery [45].

Infections of the Male Reproductive Tract

Infections of the male reproductive tract can cause inflammation, scarring, and blockages. They can also affect the quality and quantity of sperm produced. A variety of microorganisms has been identified as potential causative agents of male reproductive tract infection. These microorganisms typically establish colonies in the semen, regardless of whether their infection origin lies in the primary genital tract or the genito-urinary tract of the male. Bacterial species, specifically genital mycoplasmas, are known to infiltrate genital tracts such as *Ureaplasma urealyticum* and *Mycoplasma hominis* [46]. Pathologies such as urethritis, prostatitis, and, in certain cases, orchitis are a result of these microbial infestations. The report suggests that ureaplasmas are responsible for non-chlamydial, non-gonococcal urethritis in males [47]. Some studies have demonstrated that *M. hominis* and *U. urealyticum* do not contribute to the deterioration in sperm quality. Contrarily, in several studies, incubation with *M. hominis* showed a detrimental impact on sperm motility and morphology. Increased levels of granulocyte elastase in the seminal plasma serve as diagnostic markers for male genital tract infections, with approximately 20-30% of infertile men harboring silent genital inflammations, according to the World Health Organization (WHO) [48, 49]. Alterations in sperm attributes and apoptotic markers, seminal contamination from excess leucocytes resulting from inflammation in the male genital tract, and the generation of toxic ROS contingent on the infectious agents have all been proposed as potential contributing factors to male infertility.

Injuries to the Male Reproductive Tract

Injuries to the male reproductive tract can also cause infertility [50]. They can affect the testicles, epididymis, vas deferens, prostate gland, and urethra. Some of the common injuries that can affect the male reproductive system include:

Testicular trauma: This can be caused by a direct blow or injury to the testicles. It can cause pain, swelling, and bruising of the scrotum. It can also affect the quality and quantity of sperm produced, leading to infertility [50].

Vasectomy: This is a surgical procedure that involves cutting or sealing the vas deferens, which is the tube that carries sperm from the testicles to the urethra. It is a form of permanent contraception and can lead to infertility [51].

Prostate surgery: This is a surgical procedure that involves the removal or partial removal of the prostate gland. It can be done to treat prostate cancer, but it can also lead to infertility by affecting the quality and quantity of sperm produced [52].

Urethral trauma: This can be caused by a direct blow or injury to the urethra. It can cause pain, bleeding, and difficulty in urination. It can also affect the quality of semen produced, leading to infertility [53].

Exposure to Environmental Toxins

Environmental toxins can disrupt immune homeostasis and the immune environment of the male reproductive tract through mechanisms such as endocrine disruption, induction of OS, inflammation, epigenetic modifications, and direct toxic effects on immune cells [54 - 56]. These disruptions can impair testicular function, disrupt spermatogenesis, and potentially affect fertility [57].

Many environmental toxicants are known to have endocrine-disrupting properties. These chemicals can mimic, block, or interfere with the function of hormones in the body, disrupting the normal operation of the endocrine system. In the context of the male reproductive tract, this can negatively affect the production and function of testosterone and other gonadotropins, which are essential for normal testicular function and immune regulation within the testes [58].

Some environmental toxicants can directly affect the function and survival of immune cells, including T cells, B cells, and macrophages, which are vital for maintaining immune homeostasis [59]. This can lead to altered immune responses in the male reproductive tract.

Environmental toxins, including industrial chemicals, pesticides, heavy metals, and other pollutants, can instigate a pro-inflammatory response, which potentially leads to immune homeostasis disruption, immune cell recruitment to the testes, induction of inflammation, and consequent impairment of testicular function. Although the precise mechanism can vary depending on the toxin, a common pathway often involves the activation of the immune system and the induction of OS [9, 60].

Upon exposure, environmental toxins may be internalized by cells and instigate cellular stress responses [61, 62]. This can lead to the production of ROS, which are chemically reactive molecules containing oxygen. High levels of ROS can inflict oxidative damage on cellular components, such as lipids, proteins, and DNA, thereby disrupting normal cellular functions. In addition to direct cellular damage, ROS can serve as signaling molecules that trigger various cellular responses. Among these is the activation of the nuclear factor kappa-light-chan-enhancer of activated B cells (NF-κB) pathway. NF-κB is a protein complex that controls the transcription of DNA and plays a key role in regulating the immune response to infection [9]. OS can lead to the activation of the NF-κB pathway, which, in turn, can upregulate the expression of pro-inflammatory genes. The upregulation of these pro-inflammatory genes results in increased production of pro-inflammatory cytokines such as TNF-α, IL-1, and IL-6, as well as chemokines like monocyte chemoattractant protein-1 (MCP-1). These cytokines and chemokines are signaling molecules that can recruit various immune cells, including macrophages and neutrophils, to sites of inflammation, in this case, the testes. As immune cells infiltrate the testes, they can induce inflammation, and when this inflammation is persistent or chronic, it can lead to tissue damage [5, 9]. For example, recruited immune cells can release more cytokines and ROS, exacerbating OS and causing further damage to testicular cells. This persistent inflammation and OS may disrupt spermatogenesis and steroidogenesis, leading to impaired testicular function, reduced sperm quality, and possibly infertility [62].

Overall, the molecular mechanism involves a multi-step process, starting from the internalization of environmental toxins to the induction of OS and inflammation, recruitment of immune cells, and potential impairment of testicular function due to chronic inflammation and oxidative stress. This is a highly complex and multi-faceted process that involves many cellular and molecular players and may differ depending on the specific type of environmental toxin involved.

DIAGNOSIS AND TREATMENT OF IMMUNOLOGICAL MALE INFERTILITY

Immunological male infertility is an important subset of male fertility issues that demand higher emphasis both in research and clinical practice. The diagnosis and treatment of this type of infertility are complex and involve an understanding of the immune interaction with sperm and reproductive components.

Diagnosis of Immunological Male Infertility

The diagnosis of immunological male infertility typically involves several steps. Initial patient history and physical examination may suggest the possibility of an immune-related problem, such as previous infections, surgeries, trauma, or exposure to environmental factors that can stimulate an immune response against sperm [63].

Laboratory testing is necessary to confirm the presence of ASAs that can interfere with sperm function. The levels of these antibodies and their impact on sperm function are crucial to understanding whether they are contributing to fertility problems. These tests may include the immunobead test (IBT), mixed antiglobulin reaction (MAR) test, or enzyme-linked immunosorbent assay (ELISA) [63].

Direct Immunobead Test (IBT): This test uses immunobeads coated with antibodies that bind to human immunoglobulins. When mixed with the patient's semen, if ASAs are present, the immunobeads will attach to the sperm, allowing for visual detection and quantification under a microscope. The number of attached beads provides an indication of ASA concentration [63].

Indirect Immunobead Test: This method is used to detect ASAs in blood serum. The procedure is similar to the direct IBT, but serum instead of semen is tested [64].

Mixed Agglutination Reaction (MAR) Test: In the MAR test, latex particles coated with human immunoglobulins are added to the semen sample. The presence of ASAs will cause agglutination (clumping), which can be quantified [65].

Sperm-Cervical Mucus Interaction Test: This test assesses the ability of sperm to penetrate cervical mucus *in vitro*, a process that can be disrupted by ASAs. It is, however, less commonly used today due to the more direct ASA tests available [66].

Computer-Assisted Semen Analysis (CASA): While not specifically a test for ASAs, CASA provides detailed information about sperm movement and behavior, which can be negatively impacted by the presence of ASAs [67].

Treatment Options in Immunological Male Infertility

Previously employed therapeutic strategies for patients with specific male sperm antibodies included immunosuppression, intrauterine insemination (IUI), and conventional *in vitro* fertilization (IVF) [68].

Immunosuppression was typically designed to lower the immune response of the body and decrease the production of ASA. There are several types of immunosuppressive drugs that may be used for male infertility, including corticosteroids, azathioprine, and cyclosporine. These drugs work by suppressing the production of immune cells or by blocking their activity. However, they may also have side effects, such as increased risk of infections, liver damage, or decreased bone density. Immunosuppressive therapy is not suitable for all cases of immunological male infertility. It is typically recommended for men who have high levels of anti-sperm antibodies in their blood or semen. These antibodies may be detected through a blood test or a semen analysis. In some cases, a biopsy of the testes may also be necessary to confirm the presence of anti-sperm antibodies. However, this type of therapy is generally not recommended unless other treatment options have been exhausted, as it can have significant side effects and risks.

Assisted reproductive techniques (ART) are a range of medical interventions that aim to help couples who are struggling with infertility. ART may involve the use of medications to stimulate ovulation, IUI, or *in vitro* fertilization (IVF). In the context of male infertility, ART may also involve the use of specialized techniques to improve the quality and quantity of sperm cells. IUI and conventional IVF are aimed at facilitating the fertilization process, irrespective of the presence of ASA. However, these treatment modalities have been largely supplanted by intracytoplasmic sperm injection (ICSI). This technique entails the direct injection of a single sperm into an egg, thereby bypassing the zona pellucida, which is the outer layer of the egg that the sperm typically needs to penetrate for fertilization to occur. Consequently, ICSI appears to effectively circumvent the adverse effects associated with male ASA [68, 69]. In some cases, lifestyle changes can also be helpful in reducing the impact of immunological factors on male fertility. For example, men who smoke are more likely to have higher levels of ASAs, so quitting smoking can be helpful. Similarly, reducing alcohol consumption and maintaining a healthy weight can also be beneficial [70].

FUTURE DIRECTIONS AND RESEARCH

The last few decades have seen an explosion of research into the immunological factors that impact male infertility. While significant progress has been made in understanding how these factors work, there are still many areas that require further research. This chapter will explore the future directions and research that is currently underway in immunological male infertility.

As research delves deeper into the complex maze of the human immune system, multiple paths for future research get uncovered, especially in the area of male infertility. These investigations promise to broaden our understanding of the mechanisms at play and assist in creating successful diagnostic methods and treatments.

The ASAs, known for their substantial role in immunological male infertility, call for further exploration. We must unravel the intricacies of the impact of ASA by identifying new markers, inventing advanced diagnostic tools, and illuminating their exact molecular influence on sperm function. Simultaneously, the function of T cells and NK cells, despite being recognized as key players in male infertility, remains largely a mystery. Their exact roles demand more rigorous research, especially considering the immunological equilibrium in the male reproductive system. Inflammatory cytokines have also been linked to male infertility. However, their specific pathophysiological mechanisms are still unclear. Upcoming studies should aim to establish the associated cytokine profiles and their direct effects on sperm quality and motility. Moreover, future genomic research, including genome-wide association studies (GWAS), may reveal new genes or genetic variants associated with immunological infertility. The detrimental effects of environmental toxins on male fertility are another area to be further explored. Understanding the specific toxins involved and defining their exposure-fertility impairment relationships is crucial.

Even though the current diagnostic and treatment tools, like direct and indirect immunobead tests, mixed agglutination reaction tests, sperm-cervical mucus interaction tests, and computer-assisted semen analysis, have improved the detection of immunological male infertility, refinement and improvement are still possible. The development of novel treatment options, including the potential of immunomodulatory therapies and personalized medicine based on a patient's unique immunological profile, is of utmost importance.

Finally, considering the complexity of the role of the male immune system in fertility, longitudinal studies tracing men from pre-puberty to adulthood could provide invaluable insight into these factors' evolution and effects on fertility. In following these research paths, we can significantly enhance our understanding of immunological aspects of male infertility, leading to innovative diagnostic tools and more effective treatment strategies.

CONCLUSION

The etiology of male infertility is significantly influenced by immunological factors, thus expanding the conventional focus from only considering anatomical and physiological abnormalities. Antisperm antibodies (ASAs) are highlighted as crucial factors in male infertility, possessing the potential to disrupt sperm function and subsequently obstruct fertilization processes. The role of immune cells, such as T-cells and natural killer (NK) cells, in male infertility is underscored, as they are suggested to potentially deteriorate sperm quality and functionality. Inflammatory cytokines are pinpointed for their detrimental impact on sperm quality and motility, which may potentially lead to fertility reduction.

Genetic predisposition is acknowledged as a contributing aspect to the development of immunological factors in male infertility, indicating that certain individuals might possess increased susceptibility to these immunological complications. Reproductive tract infections or injuries are highlighted as frequent triggers for the initiation of immunological responses, which subsequently impairs male fertility. The role of environmental toxins in triggering immunological factors that result in male infertility is emphasized, thereby stressing the critical nature of lifestyle and environmental aspects in comprehending male fertility. Diagnostic methods for identifying immunological factors contributing to male infertility encompass physical examinations, semen analysis, and more specialized tests such as ASA detection*via*blood tests or immunobead binding assays. A variety of treatment modalities exist for immunological factors causing male infertility, including immunosuppressive therapy and assisted reproductive techniques. These strategies offer comprehensive solutions aimed at enhancing fertility and boosting the likelihood of successful conception for the affected individuals and couples.

REFERENCES

[1]   Vander Borght M, Wyns C. Fertility and infertility: Definition and epidemiology. Clin Biochem 2018; 62: 2-10.
       [http://dx.doi.org/10.1016/j.clinbiochem.2018.03.012] [PMID: 29555319]

[2]   Kumar N, Singh A. Trends of male factor infertility, an important cause of infertility: A review of literature. J Hum Reprod Sci 2015; 8(4): 191-6.
       [http://dx.doi.org/10.4103/0974-1208.170370] [PMID: 26752853]

[3]   Hedger MP. The Immunophysiology of Male Reproduction. Knobil and Neill's Physiology of Reproduction. Two-Volume Set 2015; 1: 805-92.

[4]   Picut CA, de Rijk EPCT, Dixon D. Immunopathology of the male reproductive tract. Mol Integ Toxicol 2017; pp. 479-539.

[5]   Dutta S, Sandhu N, Sengupta P, Alves MG, Henkel R, Agarwal A. Somatic-immune cells crosstalk in-the-making of testicular immune privilege. Reprod Sci 2022; 29(10): 2707-18.
       [http://dx.doi.org/10.1007/s43032-021-00721-0] [PMID: 34580844]

[6]   Winkler CW, Myers LM, Woods TA, *et al.* Adaptive immune responses to Zika virus are important for controlling virus infection and preventing infection in brain and testes. J Immunol 2017; 198(9): 3526-35.
       [http://dx.doi.org/10.4049/jimmunol.1601949] [PMID: 28330900]

[7]   Chakradhar S. Puzzling over privilege: How the immune system protects—and fails—the testes. Nat Med 2018; 24(1): 2-5.
       [http://dx.doi.org/10.1038/nm0118-2] [PMID: 29315300]

[8]   Dutta S, Sengupta P, Chhikara BS. Reproductive inflammatory mediators and male infertility. Chem

Biol Lett 2020; 7: 73-4.

[9]   Dutta S, Sengupta P, Slama P, Roychoudhury S. Oxidative stress, testicular inflammatory pathways, and male reproduction. Int J Mol Sci 2021; 22(18): 10043.
[http://dx.doi.org/10.3390/ijms221810043] [PMID: 34576205]

[10]   Silva AF, Ramalho-Santos J, Amaral S. The impact of antisperm antibodies on human male reproductive function: an update. Reproduction 2021; 162(4): R55-71.
[http://dx.doi.org/10.1530/REP-21-0123] [PMID: 34338216]

[11]   Gupta S, Sharma R, Agarwal A, *et al.* Antisperm antibody testing: a comprehensive review of its role in the management of immunological male infertility and results of a global survey of clinical practices. World J Mens Health 2022; 40(3): 380-98.
[http://dx.doi.org/10.5534/wjmh.210164] [PMID: 35021297]

[12]   Shibahara H, Wakimoto Y, Fukui A, Hasegawa A. Anti-sperm antibodies and reproductive failures. Am J Reprod Immunol 2021; 85(4): e13337.
[http://dx.doi.org/10.1111/aji.13337] [PMID: 32885505]

[13]   El-Sherbiny AF, Ali TA, Hassan EA, Mehaney AB, Elshemy HA. The prognostic value of seminal anti-sperm antibodies screening in men prepared for ICSI: a call to change the current antibody-directed viewpoint of sperm autoimmunity testing. Ther Adv Urol 2021; 13: 1756287220981488.
[http://dx.doi.org/10.1177/1756287220981488] [PMID: 33519975]

[14]   Duan YG, Gong J, Yeung WSB, Haidl G, Allam JP. Natural killer and NKT cells in the male reproductive tract. J Reprod Immunol 2020; 142: 103178.
[http://dx.doi.org/10.1016/j.jri.2020.103178] [PMID: 32739646]

[15]   Gong J, Zeng Q, Yu D, Duan YG. T lymphocytes and testicular immunity: a new insight into immune regulation in testes. Int J Mol Sci 2020; 22(1): 57.
[http://dx.doi.org/10.3390/ijms22010057] [PMID: 33374605]

[16]   Irez T, Bicer S, Sahin E, Dutta S, Sengupta P. Cytokines and adipokines in the regulation of spermatogenesis and semen quality. Chem Biol Lett 2020; 7: 131-9.

[17]   Zhang J, Kong DL, Xiao B, *et al.* Restraint stress of male mice triggers apoptosis in spermatozoa and spermatogenic cells*via*activating the TNF-α system. Zygote 2020; 28(2): 160-9.
[http://dx.doi.org/10.1017/S0967199419000844] [PMID: 31933449]

[18]   Liu WH, Wang F, Yu XQ, *et al.* Damaged male germ cells induce epididymitis in mice. Asian J Androl 2020; 22(5): 472-80.
[http://dx.doi.org/10.4103/aja.aja_20_21] [PMID: 31696835]

[19]   Perdichizzi A, Nicoletti F, La Vignera S, *et al.* Effects of tumour necrosis factor-α on human sperm motility and apoptosis. J Clin Immunol 2007; 27(2): 152-62.
[http://dx.doi.org/10.1007/s10875-007-9071-5] [PMID: 17308869]

[20]   Eggert-Kruse W, Kiefer I, Beck C, Demirakca T, Strowitzki T. Role for tumor necrosis factor alpha (TNF-α) and interleukin 1-beta (IL-1β) determination in seminal plasma during infertility investigation. Fertil Steril 2007; 87(4): 810-23.
[http://dx.doi.org/10.1016/j.fertnstert.2006.08.103] [PMID: 17430733]

[21]   Lampiao F, du Plessis SS. TNF-α and IL-6 affect human sperm function by elevating nitric oxide production. Reprod Biomed Online 2008; 17(5): 628-31.
[http://dx.doi.org/10.1016/S1472-6483(10)60309-4] [PMID: 18983746]

[22]   Carrasquel G, Camejo MI, Michelangeli F, Ruiz MC. IFN-gamma alters the human sperm membrane permeability to Ca $^{2+}$. Syst Biol Reprod Med 2014; 60(1): 21-7.
[http://dx.doi.org/10.3109/19396368.2013.833658] [PMID: 24067141]

[23]   Martínez-Prado E, Camejo Bermúdez MI. Expression of IL-6, IL-8, TNF-α, IL-10, HSP-60, anti-HS--60 antibodies, and anti-sperm antibodies, in semen of men with leukocytes and/or bacteria. Am J Reprod Immunol 2010; 63(3): 233-43.

[http://dx.doi.org/10.1111/j.1600-0897.2009.00786.x] [PMID: 20055787]

[24] Qian L, Zhou Y, Du C, Wen J, Teng S, Teng Z. IL-18 levels in the semen of male infertility: Semen analysis. Int J Biol Macromol 2014; 64: 190-2.
[http://dx.doi.org/10.1016/j.ijbiomac.2013.12.005] [PMID: 24333229]

[25] Fang Y, Su Y, Xu J, *et al.* Varicocele-mediated male infertility: From the perspective of testicular immunity and inflammation. Front Immunol 2021; 12: 729539.
[http://dx.doi.org/10.3389/fimmu.2021.729539] [PMID: 34531872]

[26] Schuppe HC, Pilatz A, Hossain H, Diemer T, Wagenlehner F, Weidner W. Urogenital infection as a risk factor for male infertility. Dtsch Arztebl Int 2017; 114(19): 339-46.
[http://dx.doi.org/10.3238/arztebl.2017.0339] [PMID: 28597829]

[27] Zhao H, Yu C, He C, Mei C, Liao A, Huang D. The immune characteristics of the epididymis and the immune pathway of the epididymitis caused by different pathogens. Front Immunol 2020; 11: 2115.
[http://dx.doi.org/10.3389/fimmu.2020.02115] [PMID: 33117332]

[28] Karim FL, Ahmed MS, Al-Obeidi MA. The Role of Anti-Sperm Antibodies in Primary, Secondary, Immunological and Idiopathic Infertility in Men. South Asian Research Journal of Biology and Applied Biosciences 2023; 5(2): 33-40.
[http://dx.doi.org/10.36346/sarjbab.2023.v05i02.004]

[29] Höbarth K, Klingler HC, Maier U, Kollaritsch H. Incidence of antisperm antibodies in patients with carcinoma of the testis and in subfertile men with normogonadotropic oligoasthenoteratozoospermia. Urol Int 1994; 52(3): 162-5.
[http://dx.doi.org/10.1159/000282598] [PMID: 8203056]

[30] Amarin ZO, Obeidat BR. Patency following vasectomy reversal. Temporal and immunological considerations. Saudi Med J 2005; 26(8): 1208-11.
[PMID: 16127514]

[31] Miyamoto T, Minase G, Okabe K, Ueda H, Sengoku K. Male infertility and its genetic causes. J Obstet Gynaecol Res 2015; 41(10): 1501-5.
[http://dx.doi.org/10.1111/jog.12765] [PMID: 26178295]

[32] Fraczek M, Kurpisz M. Cytokines in the male reproductive tract and their role in infertility disorders. J Reprod Immunol 2015; 108: 98-104.
[http://dx.doi.org/10.1016/j.jri.2015.02.001] [PMID: 25796532]

[33] Saleh MM, Al-Wasiti E, Muslim AN, Yousif NG. Assessment of total antioxidant capacity, interferon-gamma and interleukin-6 in idiopathic infertile men. Pak J Biotechnol 2018; 15: 743-50.

[34] Mantovani A, Bussolino F, Introna M. Cytokine regulation of endothelial cell function: from molecular level to the bedside. Immunol Today 1997; 18(5): 231-40.
[http://dx.doi.org/10.1016/S0167-5699(97)81662-3] [PMID: 9153955]

[35] Rozwadowska N, Fiszer D, Jedrzejczak P, Kosicki W, Kurpisz M. Interleukin-1 superfamily genes expression in normal or impaired human spermatogenesis. Genes Immun 2007; 8(2): 100-7.
[http://dx.doi.org/10.1038/sj.gene.6364356] [PMID: 17215863]

[36] Bentz EK, Hefler LA, Denschlag D, Pietrowski D, Buerkle B, Tempfer CB. A polymorphism of the interleukin-1 beta gene is associated with sperm pathology in humans. Fertil Steril 2007; 88(3): 751-3.
[http://dx.doi.org/10.1016/j.fertnstert.2006.11.174] [PMID: 17335817]

[37] Jaiswal D, Trivedi S, Agrawal NK, Singh R, Singh K. Association of interleukin-1beta C + 3953T gene polymorphism with human male infertility. Syst Biol Reprod Med 2013; 59(6): 347-51.
[http://dx.doi.org/10.3109/19396368.2013.830234] [PMID: 24067094]

[38] Zamani-Badi T, Karimian M, Azami-Tameh A, Nikzad H. Association of C3953T transition in interleukin 1β gene with idiopathic male infertility in an Iranian population. Hum Fertil (Camb) 2017.
[PMID: 28974117]

[39] Kosova G, Scott NM, Niederberger C, Prins GS, Ober C. Genome-wide association study identifies candidate genes for male fertility traits in humans. Am J Hum Genet 2012; 90(6): 950-61.
[http://dx.doi.org/10.1016/j.ajhg.2012.04.016] [PMID: 22633400]

[40] Shi Y, Qi W, Xu Q, *et al.* The role of epigenetics in the reproductive toxicity of environmental endocrine disruptors. Environ Mol Mutagen 2021; 62(1): 78-88.
[http://dx.doi.org/10.1002/em.22414] [PMID: 33217042]

[41] Sharma A, Mollier J, Brocklesby RWK, Caves C, Jayasena CN, Minhas S. Endocrine-disrupting chemicals and male reproductive health. Reprod Med Biol 2020; 19(3): 243-53.
[http://dx.doi.org/10.1002/rmb2.12326] [PMID: 32684823]

[42] Leisegang K, Sengupta P, Agarwal A, Henkel R. Obesity and male infertility: Mechanisms and management. Andrologia 2021; 53(1): e13617.
[http://dx.doi.org/10.1111/and.13617] [PMID: 32399992]

[43] Chaudhuri GR, Das A, Kesh SB, *et al.* Obesity and male infertility: multifaceted reproductive disruption. Middle East Fertil Soc J 2022; 27(1): 8.
[http://dx.doi.org/10.1186/s43043-022-00099-2]

[44] Sengupta P, Dutta S, Alahmar AT. Reproductive tract infection, inflammation and male infertility. Chem Biol Lett 2020; 7: 75-84.

[45] Anderson R, Moses R, Lenherr S, Hotaling JM, Myers J. Spinal cord injury and male infertility—a review of current literature, knowledge gaps, and future research. Transl Androl Urol 2018; 7(S3) (Suppl. 3): S373-82.
[http://dx.doi.org/10.21037/tau.2018.04.12] [PMID: 30159244]

[46] Andrade-Rocha FT. Ureaplasma urealyticum and Mycoplasma hominis in men attending for routine semen analysis. Prevalence, incidence by age and clinical settings, influence on sperm characteristics, relationship with the leukocyte count and clinical value. Urol Int 2003; 71(4): 377-81.
[http://dx.doi.org/10.1159/000074089] [PMID: 14646436]

[47] Taylor-Robinson D. Infections due to species of Mycoplasma and Ureaplasma: an update. Clin Infect Dis 1996; 23(4): 671-84.
[http://dx.doi.org/10.1093/clinids/23.4.671] [PMID: 8909826]

[48] Zorn B, Virant-klun I, Vidmar G, Sešek-Briški A, Kolbezen M, Meden-vrtovec H. Seminal elastase-inhibitor complex, a marker of genital tract inflammation, and negative IVF outcome measures: role for a silent inflammation? Int J Androl 2004; 27(6): 368-74.
[http://dx.doi.org/10.1111/j.1365-2605.2004.00500.x] [PMID: 15595956]

[49] Rowe P, Comhaire F, Hargreave T, Mahmoud A. Objective criteria for diagnostic categories in the standardized management of male infertility: male accessory gland infection (MAGI) WHO Manual for the Standardized Investigation, Diagnosis and Management of the Infertile Male. Cambridge: World Health Organization, Cambridge University Press 2000; pp. 52-4.

[50] Cito G, Sforza S, Gemma L, *et al.* Infertility case presentation in Zinner syndrome: Can a long-lasting seminal tract obstruction cause secretory testicular injury? Andrologia 2019; 51(11): e13436.
[http://dx.doi.org/10.1111/and.13436] [PMID: 31589772]

[51] Andino JJ, Gonzalez DC, Dupree JM, Marks S, Ramasamy R. Challenges in completing a successful vasectomy reversal. Andrologia 2021; 53(6): e14066.
[http://dx.doi.org/10.1111/and.14066] [PMID: 33866579]

[52] Fuchkar Z. Sonography in Male Infertility Ultrasound and Infertility. CRC Press 2020; pp. 189-206.

[53] Revenig L, Leung A, Hsiao W. Ejaculatory physiology and pathophysiology: assessment and treatment in male infertility. Transl Androl Urol 2014; 3(1): 41-9.
[PMID: 26816751]

[54] Liu MY, Leu SF, Yang HY, Huang BM. Inhibitory mechanisms of lead on steroidogenesis in MA-10

mouse Leydig tumor cells. Arch Androl 2003; 49(1): 29-38.
[http://dx.doi.org/10.1080/225-01485010290031556] [PMID: 12647776]

[55]   Anyanwu BO, Orisakwe OE. Current mechanistic perspectives on male reproductive toxicity induced by heavy metals. J Environ Sci Health Part C Environ Carcinog Ecotoxicol Rev 2020; 38(3): 204-44.
[http://dx.doi.org/10.1080/26896583.2020.1782116] [PMID: 32648503]

[56]   Choudhury BP, Roychoudhury S, Sengupta P, Toman R, Dutta S, Kesari KK. Arsenic-Induced Sex Hormone Disruption: An Insight into Male Infertility Oxidative Stress and Toxicity in Reproductive Biology and Medicine. Springer 2022; pp. 83-95.

[57]   Wijesekara GUS, Fernando DMS, Wijerathna S, Bandara N. Environmental and occupational exposures as a cause of male infertility: A caveat. Ceylon Med J 2015; 60(2): 52-6.
[http://dx.doi.org/10.4038/cmj.v60i2.7090] [PMID: 26132184]

[58]   Dutta S, Sengupta P, Bagchi S, *et al.* Reproductive toxicity of combined effects of endocrine disruptors on human reproduction. Front Cell Dev Biol 2023; 11: 1162015.
[http://dx.doi.org/10.3389/fcell.2023.1162015] [PMID: 37250900]

[59]   Bahadar H, Abdollahi M, Maqbool F, Baeeri M, Niaz K. Mechanistic overview of immune modulatory effects of environmental toxicants. Inflamm Allergy Drug Targets 2015; 13(6): 382-6.
[http://dx.doi.org/10.2174/1871528114666150529103003] [PMID: 26021322]

[60]   Wong EWP, Cheng CY. Impacts of environmental toxicants on male reproductive dysfunction. Trends Pharmacol Sci 2011; 32(5): 290-9.
[http://dx.doi.org/10.1016/j.tips.2011.01.001] [PMID: 21324536]

[61]   Bisht S, Faiq M, Tolahunase M, Dada R. Oxidative stress and male infertility. Nat Rev Urol 2017; 14(8): 470-85.
[http://dx.doi.org/10.1038/nrurol.2017.69] [PMID: 28508879]

[62]   Franco R, Sánchez-Olea R, Reyes-Reyes EM, Panayiotidis MI. Environmental toxicity, oxidative stress and apoptosis: Ménage à Trois. Mutat Res Genet Toxicol Environ Mutagen 2009; 674(1-2): 3-22.
[http://dx.doi.org/10.1016/j.mrgentox.2008.11.012] [PMID: 19114126]

[63]   McLachlan RI. Basis, diagnosis and treatment of immunological infertility in men. J Reprod Immunol 2002; 57(1-2): 35-45.
[http://dx.doi.org/10.1016/S0165-0378(02)00014-1] [PMID: 12385832]

[64]   Bohring C, Krause W. The intra- and inter-assay variation of the indirect mixed antiglobulin reaction test: is a quality control suitable? Hum Reprod 1999; 14(7): 1802-5.
[http://dx.doi.org/10.1093/humrep/14.7.1802] [PMID: 10402393]

[65]   Rajah SV, Parslow JM, Howell RJS, Hendry WF. Comparison of mixed antiglobulin reaction and direct immunobead test for detection of sperm-bound antibodies in subfertile males. Fertil Steril 1992; 57(6): 1300-3.
[http://dx.doi.org/10.1016/S0015-0282(16)55091-2] [PMID: 1601154]

[66]   Eggert-Kruse W, Hofsäß A, Haury E, Tilgen W, Gerhard I, Runnebaum B. Relationship between local anti-sperm antibodies and sperm–mucus interaction *in vitro* and *in vivo*. Hum Reprod 1991; 6(2): 267-76.
[http://dx.doi.org/10.1093/oxfordjournals.humrep.a137320] [PMID: 2056025]

[67]   Amann RP, Waberski D. Computer-assisted sperm analysis (CASA): Capabilities and potential developments. Theriogenology 2014; 81: 5-17. e3.

[68]   Leathersich S, Hart RJ. Immune infertility in men. Fertil Steril 2022; 117(6): 1121-31.
[http://dx.doi.org/10.1016/j.fertnstert.2022.02.010] [PMID: 35367058]

[69]   Shibahara H. Assisted Reproductive Technology (ART) as A Treatment for Infertile Men with ASA Gamete Immunology. Springer 2022; pp. 155-61.

[70]   Brannigan RE. Male reproductive immunology. An introduction to male reproductive medicine 2011; 84

[http://dx.doi.org/10.1017/CBO9780511736254.006]

Inflammation-oxidative Stress Loop in Male Infertility

Abstract: An intricate relationship exists between inflammation and oxidative stress, a connection that has profound implications for male infertility. The objective of this chapter is to delineate the molecular and cellular mechanisms underpinning the loop between inflammation and oxidative stress (OS), emphasizing its crucial role in the pathophysiology of male reproductive dysfunction. This relationship is depicted as a self-perpetuating cycle in which inflammatory processes induce OS, which in turn amplifies the inflammatory response. A comprehensive analysis of the various mediators involved in this condition is performed, encompassing reactive oxygen species (ROS), cytokines, and transcription factors. This examination aims to describe the synergistic interactions that contribute to the exacerbation of this disorder. Furthermore, the chapter accentuates the potential therapeutic value of targeting these specific pathways, uncovering promising routes for intervention in male infertility. By elucidating the multifaceted interactions and consequences of this loop, this work contributes significantly to the broader comprehension of male reproductive health. It sets the foundation for the emergence of innovative diagnostic and therapeutic methodologies. By explicitly drawing a connection between inflammation, OS, and male infertility, the authors not only enhance the current understanding but also guide the direction for future research in the field. This, in turn, fosters the creation and refinement of novel strategies to address this complex and often misunderstood medical issue. The implications of this research may, therefore, reach far beyond the immediate subject, offering valuable insights for the broader scientific and medical communities.

Keywords: Andrology, Antioxidants, Apoptosis, Assisted Reproductive Techniques, Cytokines, DNA Damage, Free Radicals, Inflammation, Inflammatory Mediators, Interferons, Lipid Peroxidation, Male Infertility, Male Reproductive Health, Oxidative Stress, Reactive Oxygen Species, Reductive Stress, Semen Quality, Sperm DNA Fragmentation, Sperm Motility, Spermatozoa.

INTRODUCTION

Infertility is a complex condition that affects many couples worldwide, and it is estimated that up to 15% of couples are affected by this issue. Although infertility affects both men and women, male infertility accounts for almost 50% of all infertility cases [1]. In recent years, studies have shown that oxidative stress and inflammation play a crucial role in male infertility. Inflammation and oxidative stress are two interconnected mechanisms that have a significant impact on sperm quality, and understanding this loop can help in the diagnosis and treatment of male infertility [2 - 4].

Oxidative stress is defined as the imbalance between the production of reactive oxygen species (ROS) and the ability of the body to detoxify them [5]. These ROS include free radicals such as superoxide anion, hydroxyl radicals, and hydrogen peroxide, which can cause damage to cells and tissues in the body. The body has natural defense mechanisms to counteract the harmful effects of ROS, such as antioxidants, which neutralize the ROS and prevent cellular damage [5]. Inflammation is a response of the immune system to a threat or injury, and it is characterized by the activation of immune cells, such as macrophages and neutrophils, which release cytokines and chemokines. Both oxidative stress and inflammation can affect sperm quality and lead to male infertility [6]. Inflammation can lead to the activation of immune cells in the male reproductive tract, which can release ROS and cause oxidative stress. Oxidative stress can damage sperm DNA, lipids, and proteins, leading to decreased sperm motility, morphology, and count. Studies have shown that men with infertility have higher levels of ROS in their semen and decreased antioxidant capacity, which suggests that oxidative stress plays a significant role in male infertility [2].

Inflammation can also affect sperm quality by altering the blood-testis barrier, which separates the developing sperm cells from the blood supply. This barrier is critical for protecting the developing sperm cells from immune cells, which can recognize them as foreign and attack them. Inflammation can disrupt this barrier and allow immune cells to enter the testes, where they can release ROS and cause oxidative stress. This can lead to testicular damage and decreased sperm production. Moreover, inflammation can also affect the hormonal balance in men, which can further impact fertility [7]. Inflammation can lead to the activation of the hypothalamic-pituitary-adrenal (HPA) axis, which can cause an increase in cortisol levels. Cortisol is a stress hormone that can affect the production of testosterone, which is essential for sperm production. High levels of cortisol can lead to decreased testosterone production, which can lead to decreased sperm count and motility [8].

Understanding the inflammation-oxidative stress loop in male infertility is crucial for developing effective diagnostic and treatment strategies. Several studies have shown that antioxidant therapy can improve sperm quality in men with infertility. Antioxidant supplements such as vitamin C, vitamin E, and coenzyme Q10 have been shown to reduce ROS levels and improve sperm motility, morphology, and count. In addition, anti-inflammatory therapy, such as nonsteroidal anti-inflammatory drugs (NSAIDs), can reduce inflammation in the male reproductive tract and improve sperm quality [9 - 11]. Thus, oxidative stress and inflammation are two interconnected mechanisms that play a significant role in male infertility. Understanding the inflammation-oxidative stress loop is essential for developing effective diagnostic and treatment strategies for male infertility. Antioxidant and anti-inflammatory therapies have shown promise in improving sperm quality in men with infertility. Further research is needed to identify the underlying causes of inflammation and oxidative stress in male infertility and develop targeted therapies to address these issues.

INFLAMMATION AND OXIDATIVE STRESS

Definition of Inflammation and Oxidative Stress

Inflammation is a complex biological process that is triggered by the body's immune system in response to tissue damage, infection, or other harmful stimuli. The process involves the activation of white blood cells, cytokines, and other signaling molecules that work together to clear the affected area of the harmful agent and promote tissue healing. While inflammation is a critical defense mechanism, chronic inflammation can be harmful and has been linked to various health problems, including heart disease, cancer, and autoimmune disorders [12]. Oxidative stress, on the other hand, refers to an imbalance between the production of ROS and the body's ability to detoxify them. ROS are highly reactive molecules that are generated during normal cellular metabolism, and their production is further increased by various external factors, such as exposure to radiation, toxins, and pollutants. When the production of ROS exceeds the antioxidant defense mechanisms, it can lead to damage to cellular structures, including DNA, lipids, and proteins [13]. This, in turn, can cause inflammation, tissue damage, and a range of health problems [4].

How are they Connected?

Inflammation and oxidative stress are closely connected processes that can both promote and exacerbate each other. For example, inflammation can trigger the production of ROS by activating immune cells and promoting cellular metabolism. Similarly, oxidative stress can activate the immune system and trigger inflammation by damaging cellular structures and releasing signaling molecules. This reciprocal relationship between inflammation and oxidative stress is known as oxidative inflammation and is believed to play a crucial role in the development and progression of various health issues [14]. In the context of male fertility, oxidative stress, and inflammation can have significant impacts on the production and quality of sperm. The testes, where sperm are produced, are highly susceptible to oxidative stress due to their high metabolic activity and exposure to free radicals generated during sperm production. This can lead to DNA damage, lipid peroxidation, and impaired mitochondrial function, all of which can contribute to reduced sperm count and quality [15].

The Effects of Inflammation and Oxidative Stress on Male Fertility

Inflammation and oxidative stress are two interconnected phenomena that can have a profound impact on male fertility. Inflammation is the natural response to infection, injury, or irritation. It involves the activation of the immune system and the release of various molecules, such as cytokines and chemokines, that promote inflammation and attract immune cells to the site of injury or infection [14]. While inflammation is essential for fighting infections and healing injuries, it can also become chronic and contribute to various health problems, including male infertility [15]. Oxidative stress, on the other hand, can cause damage to sperm cells, impairing their motility, morphology, and fertilizing ability [16]. The effects of inflammation and oxidative stress on male fertility can be far-reaching and complex. Here are some of the most significant ways in which these two phenomena can impact male reproductive health:

Testicular damage: Chronic inflammation and oxidative stress can cause damage to the testicles, the primary site of sperm production in males. This damage can impair the function of Leydig cells, which are responsible for producing testosterone, and Sertoli cells, which support the maturation of sperm cells. As a result, men with chronic inflammation and oxidative stress may experience reduced sperm counts, motility, and morphology [15].

Hormonal imbalances: Inflammation and oxidative stress can disrupt the delicate balance of hormones that regulate male fertility. For example, chronic inflammation can increase the production of estrogen, a female hormone that can interfere with testosterone production and sperm development [17]. Similarly, oxidative stress can impair the function of the pituitary gland, which produces luteinizing hormone (LH) and follicle-stimulating hormone (FSH), two hormones that are crucial for sperm production and maturation [18].

Erectile dysfunction: Inflammation and oxidative stress can also contribute to erectile dysfunction, a condition in which a man is unable to achieve or maintain an erection sufficient for sexual intercourse. Inflammation can cause damage to the endothelial cells that line the blood vessels in the penis, impairing blood flow and reducing the ability to achieve an erection. Similarly, oxidative stress can cause damage to the nerves that control the blood vessels, leading to impaired nerve signaling and reduced blood flow [19, 20].

DNA damage: Both inflammation and oxidative stress can cause damage to the DNA in sperm cells, leading to mutations and chromosomal abnormalities. These genetic changes can impair the ability of sperm cells to fertilize an egg, leading to infertility or miscarriages. Moreover, these mutations can be passed on to offspring, leading to a higher risk of birth defects and genetic disorders [21, 22].

Immune system dysfunction: Chronic inflammation and oxidative stress can also impair the function of the immune system, leading to an increased risk of infections and autoimmune diseases [23]. In the male reproductive system, this can contribute to prostatitis, a condition in which the prostate gland becomes inflamed and swollen, leading to pain and discomfort. Prostatitis can also impair the function of the prostate gland, which produces seminal fluid that nourishes and protects sperm cells [15].

Thus, inflammation and oxidative stress are two interconnected phenomena that can have a profound impact on male fertility. Chronic inflammation and oxidative stress can cause damage to the testicles, disrupt hormonal balance, contribute to erectile dysfunction, cause DNA damage, and impair immune system function [18, 24].

INFLAMMATION-OXIDATIVE STRESS LOOP IN MALE INFERTILITY

Inflammation and oxidative stress have been recognized as key players in the development of many diseases, including male infertility [2, 14]. The role of the inflammation-oxidative stress loop in male infertility has been a topic of much research in recent years.

The Role of Inflammation-Oxidative Stress Loop in Male Infertility

Inflammation and oxidative stress are two distinct but closely related processes that contribute to the development of male infertility. Inflammation is a response to cellular damage or infection that involves the release of inflammatory mediators, such as cytokines, chemokines, and growth factors. These mediators attract immune cells to the site of damage or infection, where they attempt to eliminate the cause of the inflammation. Oxidative stress, on the other hand, is a process that involves the production of reactive oxygen species (ROS) in the body. ROS are highly reactive molecules that can cause cellular damage by oxidizing lipids, proteins, and DNA. The body has mechanisms to neutralize ROS, but when the production of ROS exceeds the capacity of these mechanisms, oxidative stress occurs [14].

Inflammation and oxidative stress are closely related because inflammation can lead to the production of ROS, and oxidative stress can trigger inflammation. This creates a vicious cycle of inflammation-oxidative stress loop that can contribute to the development of male infertility [4]. The inflammation-oxidative stress loop can be initiated by a variety of factors, including infection, trauma, exposure to environmental toxins, and lifestyle factors such as diet and exercise. These factors can cause damage to sperm cells and trigger an inflammatory response that leads to the production of ROS. The ROS, in turn, can cause further damage to the sperm cells and trigger more inflammation, creating a cycle of inflammation-oxidative stress loop that can ultimately lead to male infertility [25]. Reductive stress, distinct from oxidative stress, is an emerging concern in the study of inflammation-induced male infertility. It arises from an overaccumulation of reducing equivalents, specifically NADH, creating an imbalance in the cellular redox state. Unlike oxidative stress, where an overabundance of reactive oxygen species damages cellular components, reductive stress leads to a surplus of reducing molecules, compromising cellular function. This altered redox balance can exacerbate inflammation and disrupt the normal physiology of sperm cells. The spermatozoa's motility and integrity may be impaired, leading to a diminished fertilizing capacity. Therefore, both oxidative and reductive stress create a complex interplay in the cycle of inflammation and oxidative stress, thereby impacting male fertility. Understanding this duality offers a more comprehensive perspective on the multifaceted factors contributing to inflammation-induced male infertility (Fig. **8**).

How it Affects Sperm Function?

The inflammation-oxidative stress loop can have a significant impact on sperm function, which can contribute to male infertility. Sperm are highly sensitive to oxidative stress, and the production of ROS can damage the structure and function of the sperm cells. The production of ROS can damage the plasma membrane of the sperm, which is essential for maintaining the integrity of the cell. When the plasma membrane is damaged, it can lead to the leakage of intracellular components, such as enzymes and metabolites, which can further contribute to the cycle of inflammation-oxidative stress loop. ROS can also damage the DNA of the sperm, which can lead to chromosomal abnormalities and reduce the fertility potential of the sperm. DNA damage can also lead to the formation of sperm with abnormal morphology, which can further reduce the fertility potential of the sperm [2, 25]. In addition to the direct impact of ROS on sperm function, inflammation can also contribute to male infertility by disrupting the blood-testis barrier. The blood-testis barrier is a specialized structure that separates the germ cells from the blood vessels, and it is essential for the development of healthy sperm. Inflammation can disrupt the blood-testis barrier, allowing immune cells and inflammatory mediators to enter the testes and directly damage the sperm cells [7].

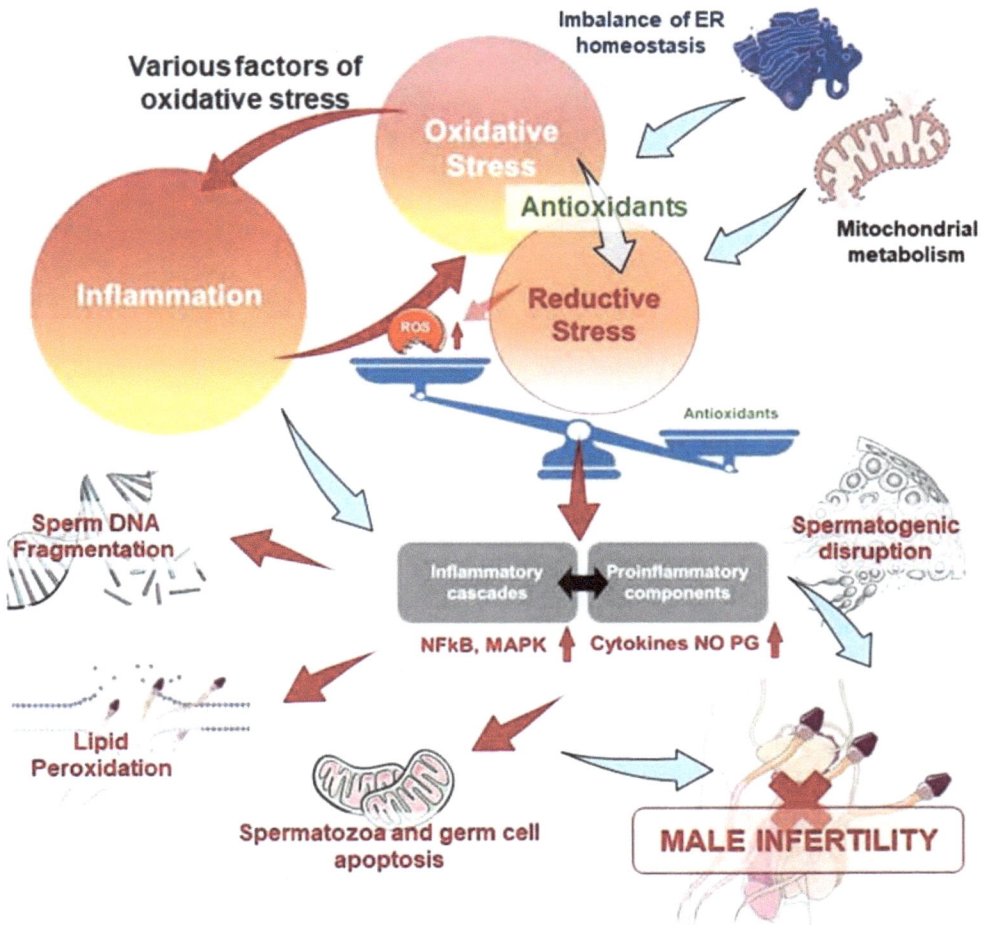

Fig. (8). Schematic Representation of the Inflammation-Redox Loop in Male Infertility. The diagram illustrates the cyclical relationship among inflammation, oxidative stress, and reductive stress, highlighting key mediators and pathways that contribute to male reproductive dysfunctions. ER, endoplasmic reticulum; ROS, reactive oxygen species; NFkβ, Nuclear factor kappa B; NO, nitric oxide; PG, prostaglandins.

CAUSES OF INFLAMMATION-OXIDATIVE STRESS LOOP IN MALE INFERTILITY

Environmental Factors

Exposure to Chemicals: Environmental factors such as exposure to chemicals, toxins, and pollutants have been linked to male infertility. Chemicals found in pesticides, herbicides, and industrial chemicals have been shown to disrupt the endocrine system, which plays a crucial role in the regulation of male reproductive function. Exposure to these chemicals can lead to the production of reactive oxygen species (ROS) and inflammation in the male reproductive system, which can damage sperm DNA, leading to decreased sperm quality and quantity [26]. For example, studies have found that exposure to organochlorine pesticides, such as DDT and PCBs, can lead to increased oxidative stress and decreased sperm motility and viability [27].

Air Pollution: Air pollution is another environmental factor that has been linked to male infertility. Air pollution is a complex mixture of gases, particles, and organic compounds, and exposure to these pollutants can lead to the production of ROS and inflammation in the male reproductive system [28]. Studies have found that exposure to air pollution can lead to decreased sperm quality and quantity, as well as increased levels of oxidative stress in the semen [29].

Heavy Metals: Heavy metals such as lead, cadmium, and mercury have also been linked to male infertility. Exposure to these metals can lead to the production of ROS and inflammation in the male reproductive system, which can damage sperm DNA and lead to decreased sperm quality and quantity [26]. For example, studies have found that exposure to lead can lead to decreased sperm motility and viability, as well as increased levels of oxidative stress in the semen [30].

Lifestyle Choices

Diet: Diet plays a crucial role in the development of the inflammation-oxidative stress loop in male infertility. A diet high in processed foods, sugar, and unhealthy fats can lead to the production of ROS and inflammation in the body, including the male reproductive system. On the other hand, a diet rich in antioxidants, such as fruits, vegetables, and nuts, can help to reduce oxidative stress and inflammation in the body [31]. Studies have found that men who consume a diet rich in antioxidants have improved sperm quality and quantity, as well as decreased levels of oxidative stress in the semen [32].

Smoking: Smoking is a major lifestyle choice that can contribute to the development of the inflammation-oxidative stress loop in male infertility. Smoking has been shown to increase the production of ROS in the body, including the male reproductive system, leading to increased levels of oxidative stress and inflammation [33]. Studies have found that smoking can lead to decreased sperm quality and quantity, as well as increased levels of oxidative stress in the semen [34, 35].

Alcohol: Alcohol consumption is another lifestyle choice that can contribute to the development of the inflammation-oxidative stress loop in male infertility. Alcohol consumption has been shown to increase the production of ROS in the body, including the male reproductive system, leading to increased levels of oxidative stress and inflammation. Studies have found that alcohol consumption can lead to decreased sperm quality and quantity, as well as increased levels of oxidative stress in the semen [36].

Genetics

Genetics plays a significant role in male infertility. A genetic mutation or an abnormality can cause a disturbance in the natural balance of hormones and chemicals in the body, leading to inflammation and oxidative stress [37]. One of the genetic conditions that cause male infertility is Klinefelter syndrome. It is a genetic disorder that affects the sex chromosomes, resulting in the presence of an extra X chromosome in males. This condition can cause hormonal imbalances, leading to testicular failure and low sperm count. Another genetic condition that can cause male infertility is Y-chromosome microdeletion. In this condition, small segments of the Y chromosome are missing, leading to poor sperm production and impaired sperm motility. This condition can be diagnosed through genetic testing [38, 39].

Additionally, some genetic mutations can cause oxidative stress and inflammation in the body, leading to male infertility. For instance, the MTHFR gene mutation can affect the ability of the body to process folic acid, leading to elevated homocysteine levels and oxidative stress [40]. This mutation has been linked to male infertility, as high levels of homocysteine can damage the sperm DNA. Moreover, some genetic polymorphisms, such as those in the glutathione S-transferase (GST) gene family, can also affect the ability of the body to detoxify harmful substances, leading to oxidative stress and inflammation [41]. This, in turn, can cause sperm damage and male infertility.

Medical Conditions

Certain medical conditions can also cause the inflammation-oxidative stress loop in male infertility. These conditions can affect the testes, sperm production, or hormonal balance, leading to oxidative stress and inflammation. One of the medical conditions that can cause male infertility is varicocele [42]. It is a condition in which the veins that drain blood from the testicles become enlarged and twisted, leading to poor blood flow and heat accumulation in the testicles. This can cause oxidative stress, inflammation, and sperm DNA damage. Moreover, infections such as epididymitis and orchitis can cause inflammation in the testicles, leading to sperm damage and male infertility. Sexually transmitted infections (STIs) such as chlamydia and gonorrhea can also cause inflammation and scarring in the reproductive system, leading to infertility [15]. Additionally, autoimmune diseases such as systemic lupus erythematosus (SLE) and rheumatoid arthritis (RA) can cause inflammation and oxidative stress in the body, leading to sperm damage and male infertility [43]. These conditions can affect the testes, hormonal balance, and immune system, leading to impaired sperm production and motility.

Furthermore, some medical treatments, such as chemotherapy and radiation therapy, can also cause inflammation and oxidative stress, leading to male infertility [44, 45]. These treatments can damage the DNA of the sperm cells and impair their function.

TREATMENT AND PREVENTION OF INFLAMMATION-OXIDATIVE STRESS LOOP IN MALE INFERTILITY

Lifestyle Changes

Exercise: Regular exercise is an effective way to reduce inflammation and oxidative stress. Exercise promotes the production of antioxidants, which help reduce oxidative stress. It also helps to regulate the immune system, which can reduce inflammation. Exercise also improves blood flow to the testicles, which can improve sperm production. Men should aim for at least 30 minutes of moderate exercise per day [46].

Sleep: Sleep is essential for reducing inflammation and oxidative stress. Lack of sleep can increase inflammation and oxidative stress. Men should aim for at least 7-8 hours of sleep per night [47].

Stress Management: Chronic stress can lead to inflammation and oxidative stress. Men should practice stress-management techniques such as meditation, yoga, or deep breathing to reduce stress [48].

Avoiding Toxins: Toxins such as tobacco smoke, alcohol, and recreational drugs can increase inflammation and oxidative stress. Men should avoid or limit their exposure to these toxins [27, 33, 49].

Dietary Modifications

Anti-inflammatory Foods: Dietary changes can help to reduce inflammation and oxidative stress. Men should focus on eating anti-inflammatory foods such as fruits, vegetables, whole grains, and healthy fats. These foods contain antioxidants and anti-inflammatory compounds that can reduce inflammation and oxidative stress [50].

Antioxidant-rich Foods: Antioxidant-rich foods can help reduce oxidative stress. Men should eat foods such as berries, dark chocolate, nuts, and seeds, which are high in antioxidants [9, 11].

Omega-3 Fatty Acids: Omega-3 fatty acids have anti-inflammatory properties and can help to reduce inflammation and oxidative stress. Men should eat foods high in omega-3 fatty acids, such as fatty fish, chia seeds, and flaxseeds [51].

Zinc: Zinc is an essential mineral for male fertility. It is involved in sperm production and testosterone synthesis. Men should eat foods high in zinc, such as oysters, beef, and pumpkin seeds [52].

Antioxidant Supplementation

Antioxidants are molecules that neutralize free radicals in the body, thereby preventing oxidative damage. Many studies have shown that antioxidants can significantly improve male fertility by reducing oxidative stress and inflammation. There are many different types of antioxidants, including vitamins C, E, and beta-carotene, which are found in fruits and vegetables [53, 54]. Additionally, there are other antioxidant supplements that have been specifically designed to improve male fertility. One of the most commonly used antioxidant supplements for male infertility is Coenzyme Q10 (CoQ10). CoQ10 is naturally produced in the body and helps convert food into energy. It is also a potent antioxidant that protects the sperm from oxidative damage. Studies have shown that supplementing with CoQ10 can significantly improve sperm count, motility, and morphology, which are all important factors for male fertility [55, 56]. Another antioxidant supplement that has been found to improve male fertility is L-carnitine. L-carnitine is an amino acid that plays a crucial role in energy production and metabolism. It is also essential for the proper functioning of the male reproductive system. Studies have shown that supplementing with L-carnitine can improve sperm count, motility, and morphology. Additionally, L-carnitine has been shown to reduce inflammation and oxidative stress in the male reproductive tract [57].

Medical Treatments

There are several medical treatments that can be used to break the inflammation-oxidative stress loop and improve male fertility. These treatments include anti-inflammatory drugs, antibiotics, and hormone therapy. Anti-inflammatory drugs such as ibuprofen and aspirin are commonly used to reduce inflammation in the body [50]. These drugs work by blocking the production of prostaglandins, which are hormones that cause inflammation. While these drugs can be effective in reducing inflammation, they should be used with caution as they can also have negative side effects, such as stomach ulcers and bleeding. Antibiotics are often prescribed to treat infections in the male reproductive system. Infections can cause inflammation and oxidative stress, which can significantly impact male fertility. Antibiotics work by killing the bacteria that are causing the infection. While antibiotics can be effective in treating infections, they should only be used when necessary, as overuse can lead to antibiotic resistance [50, 58]. Hormone therapy is another medical treatment that can be used to improve male fertility. Hormone therapy is often used to treat hormonal imbalances that can impact male fertility. For example, low testosterone levels can lead to a decrease in sperm production and quality. Hormone therapy can help increase testosterone levels, which can improve male fertility. However, hormone therapy should only be used under the guidance of a healthcare professional, as it can have negative side effects [59].

CONCLUSION

The intricate interplay between inflammation and oxidative stress has been shown to be critically involved in the decline of sperm health and functionality. There is an unending loop in which inflammation leads to the generation of ROS, which, in turn, exacerbates the inflammatory processes. This cyclical process presents a substantial risk to the production of sperm and the preservation of their structure. Acknowledging this mutual influence is crucial for understanding the fundamental disease processes at play, as well as for devising specific therapeutic strategies.

It is imperative that future research adopts a diverse set of strategies. Firstly, it is essential to create a more all-encompassing understanding of the molecular interconnections between inflammation and oxidative stress. Utilizing advanced omics techniques, such as transcriptomics, proteomics, and metabolomics, will enable a deeper exploration of the molecular agents and factors implicated in this cycle. Furthermore, a rigorous assessment of the possible anti-inflammatory and antioxidant substances that can counteract the negative impacts on male fertility is necessary. There is also a need for personalized medicine approaches that take into account genetic factors and environmental exposures, as these may facilitate more customized management of male infertility.

Lastly, the conduction of translational research and clinical trials is indispensable for determining the effectiveness and safety of innovative treatments aimed at breaking the cycle between inflammation and oxidative stress. The collective efforts of this research have the potential to usher in a revolutionary phase in the detection, management, and prevention of male infertility.

REFERENCES

[1]   Agarwal A, Mulgund A, Hamada A, Chyatte MR. A unique view on male infertility around the globe. Reprod Biol Endocrinol 2015; 13(1): 37.
[http://dx.doi.org/10.1186/s12958-015-0032-1] [PMID: 25928197]

[2]   Dutta S, Sengupta P, Slama P, Roychoudhury S. Oxidative stress, testicular inflammatory pathways, and male reproduction. Int J Mol Sci 2021; 22(18): 10043.
[http://dx.doi.org/10.3390/ijms221810043] [PMID: 34576205]

[3]   Agarwal A, Leisegang K, Sengupta P. Oxidative stress in pathologies of male reproductive disorders Pathology. Elsevier 2020; pp. 15-27.
[http://dx.doi.org/10.1016/B978-0-12-815972-9.00002-0]

[4]   Dutta S, Sengupta P, Roychoudhury S, Chakravarthi S, Wang CW, Slama P. Antioxidant Paradox in Male Infertility: 'A Blind Eye' on Inflammation. Antioxidants 2022; 11(1): 167.
[http://dx.doi.org/10.3390/antiox11010167] [PMID: 35052671]

[5]   Agarwal A, Sengupta P. Oxidative stress and its association with male infertility. Male infertility: contemporary clinical approaches, andrology, ART and antioxidants 2020; 57-68.
[http://dx.doi.org/10.1007/978-3-030-32300-4_6]

[6]   Irez T, Bicer S, Sahin S, Dutta S, Sengupta P. Cytokines and adipokines in the regulation of spermatogenesis and semen quality. Chem Biol Lett 2020; 7: 131-9.

[7]   Dutta S, Sandhu N, Sengupta P, Alves MG, Henkel R, Agarwal A. Somatic-immune cells crosstalk in-the-making of testicular immune privilege. Reprod Sci 2022; 29(10): 2707-18.
[http://dx.doi.org/10.1007/s43032-021-00721-0] [PMID: 34580844]

[8]   Viau V. Functional cross-talk between the hypothalamic-pituitary-gonadal and -adrenal axes. J Neuroendocrinol 2002; 14(6): 506-13.
[http://dx.doi.org/10.1046/j.1365-2826.2002.00798.x] [PMID: 12047726]

[9]   Agarwal A, Sekhon LH. The role of antioxidant therapy in the treatment of male infertility. Hum Fertil (Camb) 2010; 13(4): 217-25.
[http://dx.doi.org/10.3109/14647273.2010.532279] [PMID: 21117931]

[10]   Agarwal A, Finelli R, Selvam MKP, *et al.* A global survey of reproductive specialists to determine the clinical utility of oxidative stress testing and antioxidant use in male infertility. World J Mens Health 2021; 39(3): 470-88.
[http://dx.doi.org/10.5534/wjmh.210025] [PMID: 33831977]

[11]   Arafa M, Agarwal A, Majzoub A, *et al.* Efficacy of antioxidant supplementation on conventional and advanced sperm function tests in patients with idiopathic male infertility. Antioxidants 2020; 9(3): 219.
[http://dx.doi.org/10.3390/antiox9030219] [PMID: 32155908]

[12]   Schuppe H-C, Meinhardt A. Immune privilege and inflammation of the testis Immunology of Gametes and Embryo Implantation 88. Karger Publishers 2005; pp. 1-14.

[13]   Makker K, Agarwal A, Sharma R. Oxidative stress & male infertility. Indian J Med Res 2009; 129(4): 357-67.
[PMID: 19535829]

[14]   Chatterjee S. Oxidative stress, inflammation, and disease Oxidative stress and biomaterials. Elsevier 2016; pp. 35-58.
[http://dx.doi.org/10.1016/B978-0-12-803269-5.00002-4]

[15]   Sengupta P, Dutta S, Alahmar AT. Reproductive tract infection, inflammation and male infertility. Chem Biol Lett 2020; 7: 75-84.

[16]   Saleh RA, Hcld AA. Oxidative stress and male infertility: from research bench to clinical practice. J Androl 2002; 23(6): 737-52.

[http://dx.doi.org/10.1002/j.1939-4640.2002.tb02324.x] [PMID: 12399514]

[17]   Dutta S, Biswas A, Sengupta P. Obesity, endocrine disruption and male infertility. Asian Pac J Reprod 2019; 8(5): 195.
[http://dx.doi.org/10.4103/2305-0500.268133]

[18]   Darbandi M, Darbandi S, Agarwal A, *et al.* Reactive oxygen species and male reproductive hormones. Reprod Biol Endocrinol 2018; 16(1): 87.
[http://dx.doi.org/10.1186/s12958-018-0406-2] [PMID: 30205828]

[19]   Hatzimouratidis K, Amar E, Eardley I, *et al.* Guidelines on male sexual dysfunction: erectile dysfunction and premature ejaculation. Eur Urol 2010; 57(5): 804-14.
[http://dx.doi.org/10.1016/j.eururo.2010.02.020] [PMID: 20189712]

[20]   Kessler A, Sollie S, Challacombe B, Briggs K, Van Hemelrijck M. The global prevalence of erectile dysfunction: a review. BJU Int 2019; 124(4): 587-99.
[http://dx.doi.org/10.1111/bju.14813] [PMID: 31267639]

[21]   Panner Selvam MK, Sengupta P, Agarwal A. Sperm DNA fragmentation and male infertility. Genetics of Male Infertility: A Case-Based Guide for Clinicians 2020; 155-72.
[http://dx.doi.org/10.1007/978-3-030-37972-8_9]

[22]   Agarwal A, Said TM. Oxidative stress, DNA damage and apoptosis in male infertility: a clinical approach. BJU Int 2005; 95(4): 503-7.
[http://dx.doi.org/10.1111/j.1464-410X.2005.05328.x] [PMID: 15705068]

[23]   Chen J, Chen J, Fang Y, *et al.* Microbiology and immune mechanisms associated with male infertility. Front Immunol 2023; 14: 1139450.
[http://dx.doi.org/10.3389/fimmu.2023.1139450] [PMID: 36895560]

[24]   Cutolo M, Sulli A, Capellino S, *et al.* Sex hormones influence on the immune system: basic and clinical aspects in autoimmunity. Lupus 2004; 13(9): 635-8.
[http://dx.doi.org/10.1191/0961203304lu1094oa] [PMID: 15485092]

[25]   Dutta S, Sengupta P, Chakravarthi S. Oxidant-Sensitive Inflammatory Pathways and Male Reproductive Functions Oxidative Stress and Toxicity in Reproductive Biology and Medicine: A Comprehensive Update on Male Infertility-Volume One. Springer 2022; pp. 165-80.
[http://dx.doi.org/10.1007/978-3-030-89340-8_8]

[26]   Sengupta P. Environmental and occupational exposure of metals and their role in male reproductive functions. Drug Chem Toxicol 2013; 36(3): 353-68.
[http://dx.doi.org/10.3109/01480545.2012.710631] [PMID: 22947100]

[27]   Sengupta P, Banerjee R. Environmental toxins. Hum Exp Toxicol 2014; 33(10): 1017-39.
[http://dx.doi.org/10.1177/0960327113515504] [PMID: 24347299]

[28]   Jurewicz J, Dziewirska E, Radwan M, Hanke W. Air pollution from natural and anthropic sources and male fertility. Reprod Biol Endocrinol 2018; 16(1): 109.
[http://dx.doi.org/10.1186/s12958-018-0430-2] [PMID: 30579357]

[29]   Najafi TF, Roudsari RL, Namvar F, Ghanbarabadi VG, Talasaz ZH, Esmaeli M. Air pollution and quality of sperm: a meta-analysis. Iranian Red Cres Med J. 2015; p. 17.

[30]   Dutta S, Sengupta P, Bagchi S, *et al.* Reproductive toxicity of combined effects of endocrine disruptors on human reproduction. Front Cell Dev Biol 2023; 11: 1162015.
[http://dx.doi.org/10.3389/fcell.2023.1162015] [PMID: 37250900]

[31]   Sinclair S. Male infertility: nutritional and environmental considerations. Altern Med Rev 2000; 5(1): 28-38.
[PMID: 10696117]

[32]   Giahi L, Mohammadmoradi S, Javidan A, Sadeghi MR. Nutritional modifications in male infertility: a systematic review covering 2 decades. Nutr Rev 2016; 74(2): 118-30.

[http://dx.doi.org/10.1093/nutrit/nuv059] [PMID: 26705308]

[33]   Harlev A, Agarwal A, Gunes SO, Shetty A, du Plessis SS. Smoking and male infertility: an evidence-based review. World J Mens Health 2015; 33(3): 143-60.
[http://dx.doi.org/10.5534/wjmh.2015.33.3.143] [PMID: 26770934]

[34]   Okonofua F, Menakaya U, Onemu SO, Omo-Aghoja LO, Bergstrom S. A case-control study of risk factors for male infertility in Nigeria. Asian J Androl 2005; 7(4): 351-61.
[http://dx.doi.org/10.1111/j.1745-7262.2005.00046.x] [PMID: 16281081]

[35]   Chia SE, Lim STA, Tay SK, Lim ST. Factors associated with male infertility: a case□control study of 218 infertile and 240 fertile men. BJOG 2000; 107(1): 55-61.
[http://dx.doi.org/10.1111/j.1471-0528.2000.tb11579.x] [PMID: 10645862]

[36]   La Vignera S, Condorelli RA, Balercia G, Vicari E, Calogero AE. Does alcohol have any effect on male reproductive function? A review of literature. Asian J Androl 2013; 15(2): 221-5.
[http://dx.doi.org/10.1038/aja.2012.118] [PMID: 23274392]

[37]   Krausz C, Riera-Escamilla A. Genetics of male infertility. Nat Rev Urol 2018; 15(6): 369-84.
[http://dx.doi.org/10.1038/s41585-018-0003-3] [PMID: 29622783]

[38]   Vineeth VS, Malini SS. A journey on Y chromosomal genes and male infertility. Int J Hum Genet 2011; 11(4): 203-15.
[http://dx.doi.org/10.1080/09723757.2011.11886144]

[39]   Harton GL, Tempest HG. Chromosomal disorders and male infertility. Asian J Androl 2012; 14(1): 32-9.
[http://dx.doi.org/10.1038/aja.2011.66] [PMID: 22120929]

[40]   Liu K, Zhao R, Shen M, *et al.* Role of genetic mutations in folate-related enzyme genes on Male Infertility. Sci Rep 2015; 5(1): 15548.
[http://dx.doi.org/10.1038/srep15548] [PMID: 26549413]

[41]   Liu KS, Pan F, Chen YJ, Mao XD. The influence of sperm DNA damage and semen homocysteine on male infertility. Reproductive and Developmental Medicine 2017; 1(4): 228-32.
[http://dx.doi.org/10.4103/2096-2924.224910]

[42]   Jensen CFS, Østergren P, Dupree JM, Ohl DA, Sønksen J, Fode M. Varicocele and male infertility. Nat Rev Urol 2017; 14(9): 523-33.
[http://dx.doi.org/10.1038/nrurol.2017.98] [PMID: 28675168]

[43]   Chereshnev V, Pichugova S, Beikin Y, *et al.* Pathogenesis of autoimmune male infertility: Juxtacrine, paracrine, and endocrine dysregulation. Pathophysiology 2021; 28(4): 471-88.
[http://dx.doi.org/10.3390/pathophysiology28040030] [PMID: 35366245]

[44]   Schrader M, Heicappell R, Müller M, Straub B, Miller K. Impact of chemotherapy on male fertility. Onkologie 2001; 24(4): 326-30.
[PMID: 11574759]

[45]   Kesari KK, Agarwal A, Henkel R. Radiations and male fertility. Reprod Biol Endocrinol 2018; 16(1): 118.
[http://dx.doi.org/10.1186/s12958-018-0431-1] [PMID: 30445985]

[46]   Arce JC, De Souza MJ. Exercise and male factor infertility. Sports Med 1993; 15(3): 146-69.
[http://dx.doi.org/10.2165/00007256-199315030-00002] [PMID: 8451548]

[47]   Palnitkar G, Phillips CL, Hoyos CM, Marren AJ, Bowman MC, Yee BJ. Linking sleep disturbance to idiopathic male infertility. Sleep Med Rev 2018; 42: 149-59.
[http://dx.doi.org/10.1016/j.smrv.2018.07.006] [PMID: 30377037]

[48]   Sengupta P, Chaudhuri P, Bhattacharya K. Male reproductive health and yoga. Int J Yoga 2013; 6(2): 87-95.
[http://dx.doi.org/10.4103/0973-6131.113391] [PMID: 23930026]

[49] Leisegang K, Dutta S. Do lifestyle practices impede male fertility? Andrologia 2021; 53(1): e13595.
[http://dx.doi.org/10.1111/and.13595] [PMID: 32330362]

[50] Izuka E, Menuba I, Sengupta P, Dutta S, Nwagha U. Antioxidants, anti-inflammatory drugs and antibiotics in the treatment of reproductive tract infections and their association with male infertility. Chem Biol Lett 2020; 7: 156-65.

[51] Reza Safarinejad M, Safarinejad S. The roles of omega-3 and omega-6 fatty acids in idiopathic male infertility. Asian J Androl 2012; 14(4): 514-5.
[http://dx.doi.org/10.1038/aja.2012.46] [PMID: 22659579]

[52] Kumar N, Singh AK. Role of zinc in male infertility: Review of literature. Indian Journal of Obstetrics and Gynecology Research 2016; 3(2): 167-71.
[http://dx.doi.org/10.5958/2394-2754.2016.00028.X]

[53] Zhou X, Shi H, Zhu S, Wang H, Sun S. Effects of vitamin E and vitamin C on male infertility: a meta-analysis. Int Urol Nephrol 2022; 54(8): 1793-805.
[http://dx.doi.org/10.1007/s11255-022-03237-x] [PMID: 35604582]

[54] Bolle P, Evandri MG, Saso L. The controversial efficacy of vitamin E for human male infertility. Contraception 2002; 65(4): 313-5.
[http://dx.doi.org/10.1016/S0010-7824(02)00277-9] [PMID: 12020785]

[55] Alahmar AT, Calogero AE, Singh R, Cannarella R, Sengupta P, Dutta S. Coenzyme Q10, oxidative stress, and male infertility: A review. Clin Exp Reprod Med 2021; 48(2): 97-104.
[http://dx.doi.org/10.5653/cerm.2020.04175] [PMID: 34078005]

[56] Alahmar AT, Calogero AE, Sengupta P, Dutta S. Coenzyme Q10 improves sperm parameters, oxidative stress markers and sperm DNA fragmentation in infertile patients with idiopathic oligoasthenozoospermia. World J Mens Health 2021; 39(2): 346-51.
[http://dx.doi.org/10.5534/wjmh.190145] [PMID: 32009311]

[57] Mongioi L, Calogero AE, Vicari E, et al. The role of carnitine in male infertility. Andrology 2016; 4(5): 800-7.
[http://dx.doi.org/10.1111/andr.12191] [PMID: 27152678]

[58] Dutta S, Sengupta P, Izuka E, Menuba I, Jegasothy R, Nwagha U. Staphylococcal infections and infertility: mechanisms and management. Mol Cell Biochem 2020; 474(1-2): 57-72.
[http://dx.doi.org/10.1007/s11010-020-03833-4] [PMID: 32691256]

[59] Khourdaji I, Lee H, Smith RP. Frontiers in hormone therapy for male infertility. Transl Androl Urol 2018; 7(S3) (Suppl. 3): S353-66.
[http://dx.doi.org/10.21037/tau.2018.04.03] [PMID: 30159242]

CHAPTER 6

Common Male Reproductive Tract Infections

Abstract: The chapter offers a comprehensive overview of infections affecting the male reproductive system, including bacterial, viral, and fungal infections. These pathologies, such as prostatitis, epididymitis, and urethritis, present with varying degrees of severity and can lead to dire consequences if untreated, such as infertility, chronic pain, and an elevated risk of sexually transmitted infections (STIs) transmission. While bacterial infections are prevalent, viral infections often result in increased susceptibility to other diseases, and fungal infections, though rare, are significant. The chapter explores the factors escalating the risk of these infections, including age, unprotected sexual activities, prior history of STIs, and prostate enlargement. A thorough review of the diagnostic process is provided, emphasizing the importance of a medical history review, physical examination, and laboratory tests to ascertain the infection's type and gravity. Treatment protocols and preventive measures, including safe sex practices, routine medical screenings, and personal hygiene, are detailed. The significance of this chapter lies in its potential to guide a more robust, proactive approach to male reproductive health, contributing to overall well-being and disease control.

Keywords: Bacterial Infections, *Chlamydia trachomatis*, Epididymitis, Gonorrhea, *Herpes genitalis*, Human Papillomavirus, Male Urogenital Diseases, Mycoplasma Infections, Orchitis, Prostatitis, Reproductive Tract Infections, Sexual Health, Sexually Transmitted Diseases, Testicular Diseases, Trichomonas Infections, Ureaplasma Infections, *Ureaplasma urealyticum*, Urethritis, Urinary Tract Infections, Urogenital Neoplasms.

INTRODUCTION

The male reproductive tract is a complex system that includes the testes, epididymis, vas deferens, seminal vesicles, prostate, and urethra. These organs work together to produce, store, and transport sperm, as well as secrete semen. Unfortunately, like any other part of the body, the male reproductive system can become infected, leading to a range of potential health problems [1]. Male reproductive tract infections (RTIs) can be caused by a variety of microorganisms, including bacteria, viruses, fungi, and parasites. These infections can be spread through sexual contact, as well as through other means, such as poor hygiene or exposure to contaminated fluids or materials [2].

Male RTIs are common health conditions that can cause significant morbidity and mortality if left untreated. RTIs can affect any part of the male reproductive system, including the testes, epididymis, vas deferens, prostate, urethra, and seminal vesicles [3]. These infections can lead to infertility, chronic pelvic pain, and even cancer if not detected and treated early. The purpose of this chapter is to explore the importance of awareness and early detection of male RTIs. Male RTIs are a major public health concern worldwide, with high rates of incidence and prevalence. According to a previous report by the World Health Organization (WHO), more than 340 million new cases of curable sexually transmitted infections (STIs) occur annually. Of these, about 131 million cases occur in men [4]. The most common STIs that affect men include chlamydia, gonorrhea, syphilis, human papillomavirus (HPV), and genital herpes. Other factors that can cause male RTIs include urinary tract infections, prostatitis, and epididymitis [4]. These conditions are often caused by bacterial infections and can lead to inflammation and pain in the reproductive tract. Awareness of male RTIs and their potential complications is crucial for early detection and treatment. The longer an infection goes untreated, the more likely it is to cause serious health problems such as chronic pain, infertility, and even cancer. In addition, some STIs can be passed on to sexual partners, increasing the risk of transmission and further complications [5]. Early detection of male RTIs is key to effective treatment and prevention of complications. Regular screening and testing for STIs is recommended for sexually active men, especially those with multiple sexual partners. Early detection can also help prevent the spread of STIs to sexual partners.

TYPES OF MALE REPRODUCTIVE TRACT INFECTIONS

Infections of the male reproductive tract can be caused by a variety of pathogens, including bacteria, viruses, and fungi. These infections can lead to significant morbidity and can have a negative impact on fertility [5].

Bacterial Infections of the Male Reproductive Tract

Prostatitis

Prostatitis is the inflammation of the prostate gland, which is a walnut-sized gland located just below the bladder in men. The prostate gland produces a fluid that mixes with sperm to form semen, which is ejaculated during sexual intercourse. Prostatitis can be caused by a bacterial or non-bacterial infection and is classified into four types: acute bacterial prostatitis, chronic bacterial prostatitis, chronic prostatitis without infection, and asymptomatic inflammatory prostatitis [6].

Acute Bacterial Prostatitis

Acute bacterial prostatitis is a severe and sudden infection caused by bacteria that enter the prostate gland through the urethra. The symptoms of acute bacterial prostatitis include a sudden onset of fever, chills, nausea, vomiting, frequent and painful urination, and pain in the lower back, groin, and genital area. Acute bacterial prostatitis requires immediate medical attention, and the treatment involves a course of antibiotics, pain relief medication, and plenty of rest [7].

Chronic Bacterial Prostatitis

Chronic bacterial prostatitis is a recurring infection caused by the bacteria that remain in the prostate gland after treatment for acute bacterial prostatitis. The symptoms of chronic bacterial prostatitis include recurrent urinary tract infections, frequent and painful urination, pain in the lower back, groin, and genital area, and pain during ejaculation. The treatment for chronic bacterial prostatitis involves long-term antibiotic therapy, pain relief medication, and lifestyle changes [8].

Asymptomatic Inflammatory Prostatitis

Asymptomatic inflammatory prostatitis is an inflammation of the prostate gland that does not cause any noticeable symptoms. This type of prostatitis is usually discovered during a routine medical examination, and the treatment is unnecessary unless the patient experiences symptoms in the future [9].

Epididymitis

Epididymitis is a medical condition characterized by inflammation of the epididymis. It can affect males of all ages, from newborns to older men, but it is most common in young and sexually active adults [10].

Causes of Epididymitis

There are several causes of epididymitis, including bacterial and viral infections, trauma, and sexually transmitted diseases. The most common cause of epididymitis is a bacterial infection, which is usually caused by bacteria that travel from the urethra or bladder to the epididymis [10]. These bacteria can be acquired through sexual contact or other means of exposure, such as catheterization or surgical procedures. STIs such as chlamydia and gonorrhea are also common causes of epididymitis. These infections are typically spread through sexual contact and can cause inflammation of the epididymis as well as other reproductive organs. In some cases, epididymitis can also be caused by a viral infection, such as mumps [11, 12]. Trauma to the testicles can also cause epididymitis, such as from a sports injury or a blow to the groin. In rare cases, certain medications or medical procedures can also lead to epididymitis [13].

Symptoms of Epididymitis

The symptoms of epididymitis can vary depending on the cause and severity of the condition. Some common symptoms include pain or discomfort in one or both testicles, swelling or tenderness in the scrotum, redness or warmth in the affected area, pain or discomfort during urination, discharge from the penis, pain during sexual intercourse, fever, or chills [13].

Diagnosis of Epididymitis

To diagnose epididymitis, your doctor will perform a physical examination and ask about your medical history and symptoms. They may also order laboratory tests, such as a urinalysis, to rule out other possible causes of your symptoms. In some cases, imaging tests such as ultrasound may be needed to confirm the diagnosis of epididymitis and to check for other possible complications, such as an abscess or torsion of the testicle [13, 14].

Treatment of Epididymitis

The treatment for epididymitis will depend on the underlying cause of the condition. If the cause is a bacterial infection, your doctor will prescribe antibiotics to help clear the infection [14]. It is important to take the full course of antibiotics as prescribed, even if your symptoms improve before the medication is finished. If the cause of epididymitis is an STI, it is also important to notify any recent sexual partners so that they can be tested and treated if necessary. In addition, it is recommended to abstain from sexual activity until the infection has cleared. To help relieve pain and discomfort, your doctor may also recommend over-the-counter pain medication such as ibuprofen or acetaminophen. Applying ice to the affected area can also help reduce swelling and discomfort. In some cases, if the infection is severe or does not respond to antibiotics, hospitalization may be necessary for intravenous antibiotics or drainage of any abscesses [13, 14].

Prevention of Epididymitis

There are several steps you can take to help prevent epididymitis, including practicing safe sex by using condoms, getting tested for STIs regularly if sexually active, avoiding sexual contact with anyone who has an active STI or has not been tested, keeping the genital area clean and dry, wearing protective gear during sports activities to help prevent trauma to the testicles [13].

Orchitis

Orchitis is a condition characterized by the inflammation of one or both testicles. The condition can result in pain, discomfort, and swelling. In severe cases, orchitis can lead to testicular atrophy or infertility. There are many possible causes of orchitis, including bacterial or viral infections, injury, or certain medical conditions. Treatment for orchitis depends on the underlying cause and may involve medication, rest, and other supportive measures [15].

Symptoms of Orchitis

The symptoms of orchitis can vary depending on the underlying cause and severity of the condition. Common symptoms of orchitis include pain and discomfort in one or both testicles, swelling and tenderness in one or both testicles, redness, and warmth in the affected area, pain or discomfort during urination, discharge from the penis, fever, and chills. In some cases, orchitis can cause other symptoms, such as nausea, vomiting, and fatigue. If you experience any of these symptoms, it is important to see a healthcare provider for an accurate diagnosis and appropriate treatment [16].

Causes of Orchitis

There are many possible causes of orchitis, including:

Bacterial or viral infections: Orchitis can result from infections caused by bacteria or viruses, such as STIs like chlamydia or gonorrhea, or viral infections like mumps [17, 18].

Injury: Orchitis can also occur as a result of injury to the testicles, such as from a sports injury or other trauma [19].

Certain medical conditions: Orchitis can sometimes occur as a complication of certain medical conditions, such as urinary tract infections or epididymitis [20].

Diagnosing Orchitis

If you experience symptoms of orchitis, it is important to see a healthcare provider for an accurate diagnosis. Health providers may perform a physical exam and ask about the patient's symptoms and medical history. They may also order tests, such as a urine test or a testicular ultrasound, to help diagnose the underlying cause of the symptoms [15, 21].

Treating Orchitis

The treatment for orchitis depends on the underlying cause of the condition. If the orchitis is caused by a bacterial infection, your provider may prescribe antibiotics to help clear the infection. If the orchitis is caused by a viral infection, such as mumps, supportive care such as rest, ice, and pain relief may be all that is needed. In some cases, hospitalization may be necessary to provide intravenous fluids and pain relief. In addition to medical treatment, there are also several supportive measures that can help relieve symptoms of orchitis. These include resting and avoiding strenuous activity, applying ice packs to the affected area to reduce swelling and pain, wearing supportive underwear or a jockstrap to help ease discomfort, and taking over-the-counter pain relief medications, such as acetaminophen or ibuprofen [22].

Preventing Orchitis

There are several steps you can take to help prevent orchitis:

Practicing safe sex: Using condoms during sexual activity can help reduce the risk of contracting STIs that can lead to orchitis.

Getting vaccinated: The mumps vaccine is highly effective at preventing mumps, a viral infection that can lead to orchitis.

Wearing protective gear during sports: If you participate in contact sports, wearing protective gear can help reduce the risk of injury to the testicles.

Treating underlying medical conditions: Treating conditions like urinary tract infections or epididymitis promptly can help reduce the risk of orchitis.

Urethritis

Urethritis is an inflammation of the urethra, the tube that carries urine from the bladder to the outside of the body. It is a common condition that can affect both men and women, although it is more common in men. Urethritis can be caused by a variety of infectious and non-infectious factors, including STIs, bacterial infections, viral infections, and chemical irritants [23, 24].

Causes

STIs are the most common cause of urethritis, accounting for about 70% of cases in men and about 50% of cases in women. The most common STI associated with urethritis is chlamydia, which is caused by the bacterium *Chlamydia trachomatis* [25]. Other STIs that can cause urethritis include gonorrhea, which is caused by the bacterium *Neisseria gonorrhoeae*, and t*richomoniasis*, which is caused by the parasite *Trichomonas vaginalis* [26]. Non-infectious causes of urethritis can include mechanical trauma, such as from the insertion of a catheter or other medical instrument, and chemical irritants, such as soaps, perfumes, and spermicides. In addition, certain medical conditions, such as reactive arthritis and Behcet's disease, can also cause urethritis [27, 28].

Symptoms

The symptoms of urethritis can vary depending on the underlying cause, but the most common symptoms include pain or burning during urination, discharge from the urethra, blood in the urine or semen, pain or discomfort in the pelvic area, itching or irritation in the genital area. In men, urethritis can also cause inflammation of the prostate gland (prostatitis), which can lead to additional symptoms such as pain during ejaculation and pain in the testicles or groin [29].

Diagnosis

The diagnosis of urethritis typically involves a physical examination, a review of symptoms, and laboratory tests to identify the underlying cause of the inflammation. During the physical examination, the healthcare provider will examine the genital area and may collect a sample of discharge from the urethra for laboratory testing. In addition, the healthcare provider may order urine tests to check for the presence of infection and blood tests to check for signs of inflammation. Laboratory tests for STIs, including chlamydia, gonorrhea, and trichomoniasis, may also be ordered. These tests may involve collecting a sample of discharge from the urethra or a urine sample or may require a blood test [29].

Treatment

The treatment of urethritis depends on the underlying cause of the inflammation. Antibiotics are typically used to treat bacterial STIs such as chlamydia and gonorrhea. In addition, a single dose of antibiotic medication may be used to treat non-gonococcal urethritis (NGU), which is an inflammation of the urethra that is not caused by gonorrhea. Antibiotics are also used to treat bacterial infections that are not sexually transmitted, such as those caused by *Escherichia coli* (*E. coli*) or other bacteria. Treatment may also include avoiding irritants such as soaps, perfumes, and spermicides. If the urethritis is caused by a viral infection, such as herpes or human papillomavirus (HPV), antiviral medications may be prescribed to manage symptoms, but there is no cure for these infections. In addition to medication, healthcare providers may recommend lifestyle changes such as abstaining from sexual activity until the infection has been cleared, avoiding irritants, and staying hydrated [29, 30].

The mechanisms of bacterial infections-induced male reproductive dysfunctions follow complex inflammatory pathways, which are often unique for each bacterium and are detailed in Chapter 7.

Viral Infections of the Male Reproductive Tract

Viral infections can exert deleterious effects on the male reproductive system, leading to a continuum of outcomes ranging from mild to severe manifestations. The comprehension of the underlying mechanisms, dynamics, and implications of these infections on fertility constitutes an emergent field of study that mandates continued scrutiny and cognizance [31].

Impact of Prevalent Viruses on Male Fertility

Pathogens such as HPV (Human Papillomavirus), HSV (Herpes Simplex Virus), HIV (Human Immunodeficiency Virus), Zika virus, and coronaviruses have been discerned to inflict consequential ramifications on male reproductive capabilities. These may culminate in conditions encompassing infertility, oncogenic transformations, and STIs. Despite the distinct characteristics of each virus, recurrent themes of cellular invasion, replication, and host interaction are discernible [32, 33].

Human Papillomavirus (HPV): HPV is a sexually transmitted virus that infects the genital area, including the penis, scrotum, and anus [34]. HPV can cause genital warts, which can be painful and itchy. Some types of HPV are also associated with the development of cancer, including bladder and penile cancer [35]. HPV infection can be diagnosed through a physical examination or by testing for the virus in a sample of tissue [36, 37].

Herpes Simplex Virus (HSV): HSV is a common sexually transmitted virus that can cause genital herpes. HSV infection can cause painful sores on the penis, scrotum, or anus [38, 39]. The virus can be spread through contact with the sores or through skin-to-skin contact during sexual activity. HSV infection can be diagnosed through a physical examination or by testing for the virus in a sample of tissue or fluid [40].

Human Immunodeficiency Virus (HIV): HIV is a sexually transmitted virus that attacks the immune system, leading to acquired immune deficiency syndrome (AIDS) [33, 41]. HIV can be transmitted through sexual contact, sharing needles or syringes, or from mother to child during pregnancy, childbirth, or breastfeeding. HIV infection can be diagnosed through a blood test.

Zika virus: The Zika virus has been linked to male infertility by affecting the testicular tissue. Infection can lead to a reduction in the size of testes and diminished sperm production, potentially resulting in impaired fertility [42]. Experimental studies have shown pathological changes in spermatogenesis due to Zika infection [43].

Coronavirus: COVID-19 causing Severe Acute Respiratory Syndrome Coronavirus 2 (SARS-CoV-2) is the most recent example of coronavirus, which may affect male fertility through direct and indirect mechanisms [44]. Direct testicular damage has been observed in some studies, potentially impacting sperm function. Indirect effects, such as febrile illness and systemic inflammation, may transiently reduce testosterone production and sperm quality, potentially affecting fertility [45 - 47]. However, there are conflicting reports as well; for example, a recent study comparing spermiograms of infertile men before and during the COVID-19 pandemic found no significant difference in the semen parameters, suggesting that while SARS-CoV-2 may have potential impacts on male fertility, the overall effect on spermiogram results in the general population may not be as pronounced as initially feared [48].

Dynamics of Viral Infections within the Male Reproductive System

The advancement of these infections entails a nuanced equilibrium between host immune defense mechanisms and viral virulence. Entry into the male reproductive system may occur through diverse modalities, including sexual transmission, hematogenous spread, and vertical transfer. Subsequent to penetration, viruses may circumvent host immunological responses, establishing infection. Certain viral species may even reside in a latent state, eluding immune detection, and reactivate under specific circumstances, leading to chronic or recurrent afflictions [1, 31, 42].

Detrimental Effects on Male Fertility

Viral infections may substantially impede male fertility through alteration of spermatogenesis, induction of inflammatory processes, and injury to reproductive tissues. These effects are not confined to specific viral entities but extend across various infections, thus constituting a significant health consideration [1, 42].

Diagnosis and Therapeutic Approaches

The detection and diagnosis of viral infections within the male reproductive tract is a multifaceted endeavor, often involving clinical examination, serological assays, polymerase chain reaction (PCR), and radiological imaging techniques. These methodologies facilitate precise identification and evaluation of the infection's extent. Therapeutic regimens predominantly focus on symptomatic management, attenuation of viral load, and inhibition of transmission, encompassing antiviral pharmacotherapy, immunomodulatory treatments, and supportive care [49].

The domain of viral infections contributing to male infertility remains a vibrant sphere of scientific inquiry. Forthcoming research aspires to furnish more profound insights into the infection dynamics, augment diagnostic accuracy, and devise more efficacious treatment modalities. A critical component of this investigative continuum includes an exploration of the long-term ramifications of these infections on male reproductive health. Concurrently, there is an escalating imperative to develop preventive protocols to protect male reproductive well-being.

Thus, viral infections occupy a significant and complex nexus in the panorama of male infertility (explored in detail in Chapter 8). The intricacies associated with these infections and their impacts on the male reproductive system necessitate unremitting investigation, surveillance, and the cultivation of novel therapeutic and preventive strategies. The focus on understanding, diagnosing, and addressing these conditions is paramount not solely for individual health but also in the context of wider public health paradigms.

Fungal Infections of the Male Reproductive Tract

Infections of the male reproductive tract due to fungi are less frequently observed than those induced by bacterial or viral pathogens, yet they may present an equivalent degree of difficulty in terms of management and treatment. Candidiasis, attributable to organisms belonging to the Candida genus, represents the most prevalent form of fungal infection within this physiological context [50]. (Refer to Chapter 9)

Candidiasis: Candidiasis is a fungal infection caused by the yeast Candida. Candida is normally present in the human body, but overgrowth of the yeast can cause infections, including thrush in the mouth and throat and vaginal yeast infections in women [51, 52]. In men, candidiasis can cause an itchy rash on the penis and scrotum. Candidiasis can be diagnosed through a physical examination or by testing a sample of the affected tissue [51].

Aspergillosis: Aspergillosis is a fungal infection caused by the mold Aspergillus. Aspergillus is commonly found in the environment, but it can cause infections in people with weakened immune systems, such as those with HIV/AIDS, cancer, or organ transplant recipients. In men, aspergillosis can cause inflammation of the testes or epididymis [53, 54]. Aspergillosis can be diagnosed through a physical examination or by testing a sample of the affected tissue.

Cryptococcosis: Cryptococcosis is a mycotic infection induced by the yeast genus Cryptococcus. This genus is ubiquitously present in environmental contexts but manifests pathologically in individuals with immunocompromised conditions, including those suffering from HIV/AIDS, malignancies, or those who have undergone organ transplantation. In males, cryptococcosis may additionally lead to inflammation of the testicular or epididymal regions [55, 56]. The diagnosis of this infection can be performed*via*clinical examination or through laboratory analysis of a sample from the infected tissue.

Individuals possessing compromised immune functions, those diagnosed with diabetes mellitus, or those who are currently undergoing therapy with broad-spectrum antibiotics exhibit an increased susceptibility to these mycotic infections [57, 58]. Clinical manifestations may include balanitis, characterized by inflammation of the glans penis, which is frequently accompanied by pruritus, erythema, and a leukorrheic discharge. Furthermore, the infection may extend to involve the prostate gland and other anatomical structures within the reproductive system [59].

Therapeutic interventions generally encompass antifungal pharmacological agents, which can be administered topically or systemically, the choice of which is contingent on the infection's severity and anatomical localization. Adherence to appropriate hygienic practices, in conjunction with prompt medical consultation upon the initial observation of indicative symptoms, is pivotal in forestalling the dissemination of the infection and the subsequent development of potential complications [59].

RISK FACTORS

The male reproductive system is a complex and delicate network of organs that is susceptible to infections. Infections of the male reproductive tract can occur due to a variety of reasons, and the risk factors for these infections are numerous.

Age

Age is an important risk factor for male RTIs. As men age, their immune system weakens, making them more vulnerable to infections [60]. The incidence of RTIs increases with age, and this is particularly true for infections of the prostate gland. Prostate infections, also known as prostatitis, are more common in men over the age of 50. This is because the prostate gland tends to enlarge with age, making it more susceptible to infection [61]. Prostate enlargement can also lead to urinary tract infections, which can further increase the risk of male RTIs.

Sexual Activity

Sexual activity is another major risk factor for male RTIs [62, 63]. This is because the male reproductive system is closely linked to the urinary tract, and sexual activity can introduce bacteria into the urinary tract and, ultimately, into the reproductive system. STIs are one of the most common types of male RTIs, and they are transmitted through sexual activity. STIs such as gonorrhea and chlamydia can cause inflammation of the urethra, which can lead to urinary tract infections and, ultimately, infections of the prostate gland. In addition to STIs, other types of infections can also be transmitted through sexual activity. For example, bacterial infections such as *E. coli* and *Klebsiella pneumoniae* can be transmitted through sexual activity and can cause urinary tract infections and prostatitis [64].

History of STIs

A history of STIs is a significant risk factor for male RTIs. Men who have had one or more STIs in the past are more likely to develop future infections [65, 66]. This is because the damage caused by STIs to the urethra and prostate gland can make these organs more susceptible to infection. STIs such as gonorrhea and chlamydia can cause inflammation of the urethra, which can lead to scarring and narrowing of the urethra. This can make it difficult for men to urinate and can increase the risk of urinary tract infections and prostatitis. In addition to STIs, other types of infections can also cause damage to the male reproductive tract. For example, infections of the prostate gland can cause scarring and inflammation, which can increase the risk of future infections [67].

Prostate Enlargement

Prostate enlargement is another important risk factor for male RTIs. The prostate gland is a small gland that is located just below the bladder and is an important part of the male reproductive system [68]. As men age, the prostate gland tends to enlarge, a condition known as benign prostatic hyperplasia (BPH). BPH can cause a number of symptoms, including difficulty urinating, frequent urination, and urinary tract infections. BPH can also increase the risk of prostatitis, a type of infection that occurs when the prostate gland becomes inflamed [69]. In addition to BPH, other conditions that can cause prostate enlargement can also increase the risk of male RTIs [70]. For example, prostate cancer can cause enlargement of the prostate gland and can increase the risk of infections of the prostate gland and urinary tract.

DIAGNOSIS AND TREATMENT

The male reproductive tract is susceptible to a variety of infections that can cause significant morbidity if left untreated. Infections of the male reproductive tract can affect the epididymis, vas deferens, seminal vesicles, prostate, and urethra and can result in symptoms such as urethral discharge, painful urination, scrotal pain, and infertility. The diagnosis and treatment of male RTIs require a thorough medical history, physical examination, and laboratory testing [71].

Medical History and Physical Examination

A detailed medical history and physical examination are the first steps in the diagnosis of male RTIs. The medical history should focus on symptoms, sexual practices, and risk factors for STIs, such as unprotected sex, multiple sexual partners, and a history of STIs. It is important to obtain a sexual history that includes the number and gender of sexual partners, the types of sexual practices, and the presence of any symptoms in the partner(s). The physical examination should include a genital examination to evaluate for signs of inflammation or infection, such as erythema, edema, tenderness, or discharge. The scrotum should be examined for swelling or tenderness, and the prostate should be evaluated for size, consistency, and tenderness on digital rectal examination (DRE). The DRE can also help identify any nodules or areas of induration that may suggest prostatitis or prostate cancer. In addition, the inguinal lymph nodes should be palpated to evaluate for lymphadenopathy, which may suggest the presence of an STI [71].

Laboratory Tests

Urine analysis and culture: A urine analysis and culture are often used to diagnose male RTIs. A clean-catch midstream urine specimen should be obtained for urinalysis and culture. The urinalysis can detect the presence of white blood cells, which may indicate an infection. The urine culture can identify the causative organism and determine the appropriate antibiotic treatment [72].

Urethral swab or urine nucleic acid amplification test (NAAT): A urethral swab or urine NAAT can be used to diagnose STIs such as chlamydia and gonorrhea. The urethral swab is obtained by inserting a swab into the urethra and rotating it to collect a sample of secretions. The urine NAAT is a non-invasive test that can detect the genetic material of the bacteria that cause chlamydia and gonorrhea. Both tests have high sensitivity and specificity and can be used to diagnose asymptomatic infections [73].

Semen analysis: A semen analysis may be recommended if infertility is a concern. A semen analysis can evaluate the quantity and quality of sperm and can identify the presence of white blood cells, which may indicate infection. A semen culture can also be performed to identify the causative organism [74].

Prostate-specific antigen (PSA) test: A PSA test is a blood test that measures the level of PSA, a protein produced by the prostate gland. Elevated levels of PSA may indicate prostate inflammation or infection but can also be a sign of prostate cancer. The PSA test is not specific for infection, but can be used to monitor the response to treatment for prostatitis or prostate infection [75].

Antibiotics and other Treatments

The use of antibiotics and other treatments is important in the management of male RTIs [76].

Antibiotics: Antibiotics are commonly used to treat bacterial infections of the male reproductive tract [77]. Antibiotics work by killing or inhibiting the growth of bacteria. The choice of antibiotics depends on the type of bacteria causing the infection, the severity of the infection, and the patient's medical history [76]. Commonly used antibiotics for male RTIs include:

Fluoroquinolones: These antibiotics are commonly used to treat bacterial infections of the prostate gland. Examples of fluoroquinolones include ciprofloxacin, levofloxacin, and norfloxacin.

Macrolides: These antibiotics are used to treat infections caused by Mycoplasma and Chlamydia. Examples of macrolides include azithromycin and erythromycin.

Tetracyclines: These antibiotics are used to treat infections caused by Chlamydia and other bacteria. Examples of tetracyclines include doxycycline and minocycline.

Aminoglycosides: These antibiotics are used to treat severe infections caused by Gram-negative bacteria. Examples of aminoglycosides include gentamicin and tobramycin.

Penicillins: These antibiotics are used to treat infections caused by Gram-positive bacteria. Examples of penicillins include amoxicillin and penicillin G.

Antibiotics are generally safe and effective in the treatment of male RTIs. However, their use can be associated with side effects such as gastrointestinal upset, allergic reactions, and the development of antibiotic-resistant bacteria [77].

Other treatments: In addition to antibiotics, other treatments can be used to manage male RTIs. These treatments include:

Antiviral medications: These medications are used to treat viral infections of the male reproductive tract, such as genital herpes and human papillomavirus (HPV) infection. Examples of antiviral medications include acyclovir and valacyclovir [78].

Antifungal medications: These medications are used to treat fungal infections of the male reproductive tract, such as candidiasis. Examples of antifungal medications include fluconazole and clotrimazole [79].

Immunomodulatory agents: These agents are used to modulate the immune response in the male reproductive tract. Examples of immunomodulatory agents include interferons and immunoglobulins [80].

Anti-inflammatory medications: These medications are used to reduce inflammation in the male reproductive tract. Examples of anti-inflammatory medications include nonsteroidal anti-inflammatory drugs (NSAIDs) and corticosteroids [77].

Surgical interventions: In some cases, surgical interventions may be required to manage male RTIs. For example, abscesses may need to be drained, and blockages in the epididymis or vas deferens may need to be removed [81].

PREVENTION

Safe Sexual Practices

Safe sexual practices are one of the most effective ways to prevent male RTIs. Sexual activity is the primary mode of transmission for many RTIs, including chlamydia, gonorrhea, syphilis, and HIV. Therefore, practicing safe sex can significantly reduce the risk of developing these infections [59, 82].

Use Condoms: Using condoms during sexual activity is one of the most effective ways to prevent male RTIs. Condoms create a physical barrier that can prevent the transmission of pathogens from one partner to another. When used correctly, condoms can reduce the risk of contracting many RTIs, including chlamydia, gonorrhea, syphilis, and HIV. It is important to note that not all RTIs can be prevented by using condoms. For example, genital herpes and HPV infections can still be transmitted even when condoms are used. However, condoms can still provide some protection against these infections by reducing the risk of skin-t--skin contact. It is also important to use condoms consistently and correctly to maximize their effectiveness. Condoms should be put on before any genital contact occurs and should be used for the entire duration of sexual activity. It is also essential to use the right size of the condom to ensure a proper fit [83].

Limit Sexual Partners: Limiting the number of sexual partners is another important strategy for preventing male RTIs. Having multiple sexual partners can increase the risk of contracting RTIs, as each additional partner increases the likelihood of exposure to pathogens. Therefore, reducing the number of sexual partners can significantly reduce the risk of developing these infections. If you choose to have multiple sexual partners, it is essential to practice safe sex with each partner. This includes using condoms and getting regular check-ups and screenings for RTIs [82].

Get Vaccinated: Vaccines can also play a significant role in preventing male RTIs [84]. Two vaccines, in particular, can protect against some of the most common RTIs:

HPV vaccine: The HPV vaccine can protect against certain types of HPV that can cause genital warts and certain types of cancer, including cervical, anal, and penile cancer. The vaccine is recommended for both boys and girls between the ages of 9 and 26.

Hepatitis B vaccine: The hepatitis B vaccine can protect against hepatitis B, a viral infection that can cause liver damage and cancer. The vaccine is recommended for all children and adults who are at risk of contracting hepatitis B.

Regular Check-ups and Screenings

Regular check-ups and screenings are an important part of preventing male RTIs. These check-ups should include a thorough physical exam, as well as testing for STIs and other potential causes of infection [82]. One of the most important screenings for men is a prostate-specific antigen (PSA) test. This blood test measures the level of PSA, a protein produced by the prostate gland, in the bloodstream. High levels of PSA can indicate the presence of prostate cancer or other prostate issues, such as prostatitis (inflammation of the prostate). Men over the age of 50 should have an annual PSA test or earlier if there is a family history of prostate cancer or other risk factors. Another important screening for men is testing for STIs. Many STIs, including chlamydia, gonorrhea, and syphilis, can cause male RTIs. These infections can lead to inflammation of the testes, epididymis, and prostate, as well as urethritis (inflammation of the urethra). Testing for STIs is typically done using a urine sample, blood test, or swab from the genital area. Men who are sexually active with multiple partners should be tested for STIs on a regular basis, as should men who have symptoms such as discharge from the penis, painful urination, or genital sores [82].

In addition to regular check-ups and screenings, men should also be aware of the signs and symptoms of male RTIs. These can include pain or discomfort in the testes or prostate, swelling or redness in the genital area, discharge from the penis, and pain or burning during urination. If any of these symptoms occur, men should see a healthcare provider as soon as possible for evaluation and treatment.

Proper Hygiene and Self-Care

Proper hygiene and self-care are also important for preventing male RTIs. Men should practice good hygiene habits, including washing the genital area regularly with soap and water, especially after sexual activity or exercise. They should also wear clean, dry underwear and avoid tight-fitting clothing that can trap moisture and create a breeding ground for bacteria and fungi. Proper self-care also includes avoiding activities that can lead to male RTIs. For example, men should avoid using recreational drugs, such as cocaine or methamphetamine, that can cause inflammation and damage to the genital area. They should also avoid activities that can cause trauma to the testes, such as contact sports or rough sex [82]. Men should also know the proper sustainable use of condom [83].

CONCLUSION

Infections in the male reproductive tract encompass a diverse array of pathologies, including prostatitis, epididymitis, and urethritis, which can be caused by bacteria, viruses, fungi, *etc*. If untreated, these can lead to adverse outcomes such as infertility, chronic pain, and an increased risk of STI transmission. Bacterial Infections are prevalent within the male reproductive system and present with varying degrees of severity. Notably, viral infections can lead to enduring consequences, such as an increased susceptibility to other diseases. Although comparatively rare, fungal infections are not without significance in affecting the male reproductive system.

The likelihood of acquiring RTIs is known to be influenced by age, engaging in unprotected sexual activities, prior history of STIs, and prostate enlargement, which escalate the risk of subsequent infections. The diagnostic process usually initiates with a meticulous review of medical history, followed by a physical examination. Laboratory tests are imperative for ascertaining both the type and gravity of the infection. Depending upon the nature of the infection, treatment may necessitate the use of antibiotics or other specific therapeutic agents.

Preventive measures, including adherence to safe sex practices, stand as a substantial means of curtailing the risk of infections [84]. Routine medical examinations and screenings serve as valuable tools for the early detection and prevention of potential complications. Maintenance of personal hygiene and diligent self-care routines further contribute to a diminished likelihood of infections. By recognizing and addressing these various aspects, healthcare providers can work towards more effective prevention, diagnosis, and treatment of male reproductive tract infections. Healthcare professionals should play a central role in imparting knowledge and raising awareness about the seriousness of RTIs and the importance of prevention and early intervention. Collectively, these approaches will promote a more robust and proactive culture of male reproductive health, which is indispensable in the broader context of public health and well-being.

REFERENCES

[1]   Le Tortorec A, Matusali G, Mahé D, *et al.* From ancient to emerging infections: the odyssey of viruses in the male genital tract. Physiol Rev 2020; 100(3): 1349-414.
[http://dx.doi.org/10.1152/physrev.00021.2019] [PMID: 32031468]

[2]   Henkel R, Solomon M. Semen culture and the assessment of genitourinary tract infections. Indian J Urol 2017; 33(3): 188-93.
[http://dx.doi.org/10.4103/iju.IJU_407_16] [PMID: 28717267]

[3]   Azenabor A, Ekun AO, Akinloye O. Impact of inflammation on male reproductive tract. J Reprod Infertil 2015; 16(3): 123-9.
[PMID: 26913230]

[4]   Organization W H. Global prevalence and incidence of selected curable sexually transmitted infections: overview and estimates 2001.

[5]   Sengupta P, Dutta S, Alahmar AT. Reproductive tract infection, inflammation and male infertility. Chemical Biology Letters 2020; 7: 75-84.

[6]   Khan FU, Ihsan AU, Khan HU, *et al.* Comprehensive overview of prostatitis. Biomed Pharmacother 2017; 94: 1064-76.
[http://dx.doi.org/10.1016/j.biopha.2017.08.016] [PMID: 28813783]

[7]   Coker TJ, Dierfeldt DM. Acute bacterial prostatitis: diagnosis and management. Am Fam Physician 2016; 93(2): 114-20.
[PMID: 26926407]

[8]   Gill BC, Shoskes DA. Bacterial prostatitis. Curr Opin Infect Dis 2016; 29(1): 86-91.
[http://dx.doi.org/10.1097/QCO.0000000000000222] [PMID: 26555038]

[9]   Taoka R, Kakehi Y. The influence of asymptomatic inflammatory prostatitis on the onset and progression of lower urinary tract symptoms in men with histologic benign prostatic hyperplasia. Asian J Urol 2017; 4(3): 158-63.
[http://dx.doi.org/10.1016/j.ajur.2017.02.004] [PMID: 29264225]

[10]   Zhao H, Yu C, He C, Mei C, Liao A, Huang D. The immune characteristics of the epididymis and the immune pathway of the epididymitis caused by different pathogens. Front Immunol 2020; 11: 2115.
[http://dx.doi.org/10.3389/fimmu.2020.02115] [PMID: 33117332]

[11]   Louette A, Krahn J, Caine V, Ha S, Lau TTY, Singh AE. Treatment of acute epididymitis: a systematic review and discussion of the implications for treatment based on etiology. Sex Transm Dis

2018; 45(12): e104-8.
[http://dx.doi.org/10.1097/OLQ.0000000000000901] [PMID: 30044339]

[12]   McConaghy JR, Panchal B. Epididymitis: An Overview. Am Fam Physician 2016; 94(9): 723-6.
       [PMID: 27929243]

[13]   Taylor SN. Epididymitis: Table 1. Clin Infect Dis 2015; 61 (Suppl. 8): S770-3.
       [http://dx.doi.org/10.1093/cid/civ812] [PMID: 26602616]

[14]   Wang X, Zhang Z, Fang L, *et al.* Challenges in the diagnosis of testicular infarction in the presence of
       prolonged epididymitis: Three cases report and literature review. J XRay Sci Technol 2020; 28(4):
       809-19.
       [http://dx.doi.org/10.3233/XST-200671] [PMID: 32474478]

[15]   Azmat CE, Vaitla P. Orchitis. In: StatPearls. StatPearls Publishing, Treasure Island (FL) 2023.
       [PMID: 31985958]

[16]   Schuppe HC, Pilatz A, Hossain H, Diemer T, Wagenlehner F, Weidner W. Urogenital infection as a
       risk factor for male infertility. Dtsch Arztebl Int 2017; 114(19): 339-46.
       [http://dx.doi.org/10.3238/arztebl.2017.0339] [PMID: 28597829]

[17]   Wu H, Wang F, Tang D, Han D. Mumps orchitis: clinical aspects and mechanisms. Front Immunol
       2021; 12: 582946.
       [http://dx.doi.org/10.3389/fimmu.2021.582946] [PMID: 33815357]

[18]   Bonner M, Sheele JM, Cantillo-Campos S, Elkins JM. A descriptive analysis of men diagnosed with
       epididymitis, orchitis, or both in the emergency department. Cureus 2021; 13(6): e15800.
       [http://dx.doi.org/10.7759/cureus.15800] [PMID: 34306868]

[19]   Akay S, Kaygisiz M, Oztas M, Turgut MS. Surgically confirmed intra-and extratesticular hematoma
       clinically mimicking epididymo-orchitis and radiologically mimicking traumatic torsion. Pol Przegl
       Radiol Med Nukl 2015; 80: 486-9.
       [http://dx.doi.org/10.12659/PJR.895138] [PMID: 26600877]

[20]   Street E, Joyce A, Wilson J. BASHH UK guideline for the management of epididymo-orchitis, 2010.
       Int J STD AIDS 2011; 22(7): 361-5.
       [http://dx.doi.org/10.1258/ijsa.2011.011023] [PMID: 21729951]

[21]   Silva CA, Cocuzza M, Carvalho JF, Bonfá E. Diagnosis and classification of autoimmune orchitis.
       Autoimmun Rev 2014; 13(4-5): 431-4.
       [http://dx.doi.org/10.1016/j.autrev.2014.01.024] [PMID: 24424181]

[22]   Nicholson A, Rait G, Murray-Thomas T, Hughes G, Mercer CH, Cassell J. Management of
       epididymo-orchitis in primary care: results from a large UK primary care database. Br J Gen Pract
       2010; 60(579): e407-22.
       [http://dx.doi.org/10.3399/bjgp10X532413] [PMID: 20883615]

[23]   Mändar R. Microbiota of male genital tract: Impact on the health of man and his partner. Pharmacol
       Res 2013; 69(1): 32-41.
       [http://dx.doi.org/10.1016/j.phrs.2012.10.019] [PMID: 23142212]

[24]   Holmes K K, P F Sparling, W E Stamm, P Piot, J N Wasserheit, L Corey, *et al.,* Sexually transmitted
       diseases. 2007: McGraw-Hill.

[25]   Wetmore CM, Manhart LE, Lowens MS, *et al.* Demographic, behavioral, and clinical characteristics
       of men with nongonococcal urethritis differ by etiology: a case-comparison study. Sex Transm Dis
       2011; 38(3): 180-6.
       [http://dx.doi.org/10.1097/OLQ.0b013e3182040de9] [PMID: 21285914]

[26]   Gimenes F, Souza RP, Bento JC, *et al.* Male infertility: a public health issue caused by sexually
       transmitted pathogens. Nat Rev Urol 2014; 11(12): 672-87.
       [http://dx.doi.org/10.1038/nrurol.2014.285] [PMID: 25330794]

[27]   Galadari I, Galadari H. Nonspecific urethritis and reactive arthritis. Clin Dermatol 2004; 22(6): 469-75.
[http://dx.doi.org/10.1016/j.clindermatol.2004.07.010] [PMID: 15596317]

[28]   Kirkali Z, Yigitbasi O, Sasmaz R. Urological aspects of Behçet's disease. Br J Urol 1991; 67(6): 638-9.
[http://dx.doi.org/10.1111/j.1464-410X.1991.tb15230.x] [PMID: 2070210]

[29]   Brill JR. Diagnosis and treatment of urethritis in men. Am Fam Physician 2010; 81(7): 873-8.
[PMID: 20353145]

[30]   Bachmann LH, Manhart LE, Martin DH, *et al.* Advances in the understanding and treatment of male urethritis. Clin Infect Dis 2015; 61 (Suppl. 8): S763-9.
[http://dx.doi.org/10.1093/cid/civ755] [PMID: 26602615]

[31]   Akhigbe RE, Dutta S, Hamed MA, Ajayi AF, Sengupta P, Ahmad G. Viral infections and male infertility: a comprehensive review of the role of oxidative stress. Frontiers in Reproductive Health 2022; 4: 782915.
[http://dx.doi.org/10.3389/frph.2022.782915] [PMID: 36303638]

[32]   Guo Y, Dong Y, Zheng R, Yan J, Li W, Xu Y, Yan X, Ke Y, Li Y, Xiang L. Correlation between viral infections in male semen and infertility: a literature review. Virology Journal. 2024 Jul 30;21(1):167
[http://dx.doi.org/10.1186/s12985-024-02431-w] [PMID: 39080728]

[33]   Roychoudhury S, Das A, Sengupta P, *et al.* Viral pandemics of twenty-first century. J Microbiol Biotechnol Food Sci 2021; 10(4): 711-6.
[http://dx.doi.org/10.15414/jmbfs.2021.10.4.711-716]

[34]   Goulart ACX, Farnezi HCM, França JPBM, Santos A, Ramos MG, Penna MLF. HIV, HPV and Chlamydia trachomatis: impacts on male fertility. JBRA Assist Reprod 2020; 24(4): 492-7.
[http://dx.doi.org/10.5935/1518-0557.20200020] [PMID: 32496735]

[35]   Sarier M, Usta SS, Turgut H, *et al.* Prognostic value of HPV DNA in Urothelial Carcinoma of the Bladder: A Preliminary Report of 2-Year Follow-up Results. Urol J 2021; 19(1): 45-9.
[PMID: 33931844]

[36]   Baer H, Allen S, Braun L. Knowledge of human papillomavirus infection among young adult men and women: implications for health education and research. J Community Health 2000; 25(1): 67-78.
[http://dx.doi.org/10.1023/A:1005192902137] [PMID: 10706210]

[37]   Karnes JB, Usatine RP. Management of external genital warts. Am Fam Physician 2014; 90(5): 312-8.
[PMID: 25251091]

[38]   Ross JD, Smith IW, Elton RA. The epidemiology of herpes simplex types 1 and 2 infection of the genital tract in Edinburgh 1978-1991. Sex Transm Infect 1993; 69(5): 381-3.
[http://dx.doi.org/10.1136/sti.69.5.381] [PMID: 8244358]

[39]   Lafferty WE, Downey L, Celum C, Wald A. Herpes simplex virus type 1 as a cause of genital herpes: impact on surveillance and prevention. J Infect Dis 2000; 181(4): 1454-7.
[http://dx.doi.org/10.1086/315395] [PMID: 10762576]

[40]   Omarova S, Cannon A, Weiss W, Bruccoleri A, Puccio J. Genital Herpes Simplex Virus—An Updated Review. Adv Pediatr 2022; 69(1): 149-62.
[http://dx.doi.org/10.1016/j.yapd.2022.03.010] [PMID: 35985707]

[41]   Roychoudhury S, Das A, Sengupta P, *et al.* Viral pandemics of the last four decades: pathophysiology, health impacts and perspectives. Int J Environ Res Public Health 2020; 17(24): 9411.
[http://dx.doi.org/10.3390/ijerph17249411] [PMID: 33333995]

[42]   Dutta S, Sengupta P, Chakravarthi S. Testicular immune tolerance and viral infections. Translational Autoimmunity. Elsevier 2023; pp. 169-81.
[http://dx.doi.org/10.1016/B978-0-323-85389-7.00022-3]

[43]   Ma W, S Li, S Ma, L Jia, F Zhang, Y Zhang, *et al.,* Zika virus causes testis damage and leads to male infertility in mice. Cell. 2016; 167:1511-1524. e10.
[http://dx.doi.org/10.1016/j.cell.2016.11.016]

[44]   Sengupta P, Leisegang K, Agarwal A. The impact of COVID-19 on the male reproductive tract and fertility: A systematic review. Arab J Urol 2021; 19(3): 423-36.
[http://dx.doi.org/10.1080/2090598X.2021.1955554] [PMID: 34552795]

[45]   Zhou P, X-L Yang, X-G Wang, B Hu, L Zhang, W Zhang, *et al.,* A pneumonia outbreak associated with a new coronavirus of probable bat origin. nature. 2020; 579:270-273.

[46]   Aitken RJ. COVID-19 and human spermatozoa—Potential risks for infertility and sexual transmission? Andrology 2021; 9(1): 48-52.
[http://dx.doi.org/10.1111/andr.12859] [PMID: 32649023]

[47]   Li D, Jin M, Bao P, Zhao W, Zhang S. Clinical characteristics and results of semen tests among men with coronavirus disease 2019. JAMA Netw Open 2020; 3(5): e208292-2.
[http://dx.doi.org/10.1001/jamanetworkopen.2020.8292] [PMID: 32379329]

[48]   Sarier M, Demir M, Emek M, *et al.* Comparison of spermiograms of infertile men before and during the COVID-19 pandemic. Rev Assoc Med Bras 2022; 68(2): 191-5.
[http://dx.doi.org/10.1590/1806-9282.20210935] [PMID: 35239880]

[49]   Teixeira TA, Oliveira YC, Bernardes FS, *et al.* Viral infections and implications for male reproductive health. Asian J Androl 2021; 23(4): 335-47.
[http://dx.doi.org/10.4103/aja.aja_82_20] [PMID: 33473014]

[50]   Castrillón-Duque EX, Puerta Suárez J, Cardona Maya WD. Yeast and fertility: Effects of in vitro activity of Candida spp. on sperm quality. J Reprod Infertil 2018; 19(1): 49-55.
[PMID: 29850447]

[51]   Edwards SK. Genital rash (including warts and infestations). Medicine (Abingdon) 2018; 46(6): 325-30.
[http://dx.doi.org/10.1016/j.mpmed.2018.03.005]

[52]   Karawita A, Ranawaka RR. Atlas of Dermatoses in Pigmented Skin. 2021.

[53]   Singer AJ, Kubak B, Anders KH. Aspergillosis of the testis in a renal transplant recipient. Urology 1998; 51(1): 119-21.
[http://dx.doi.org/10.1016/S0090-4295(97)00466-4] [PMID: 9457303]

[54]   Zhichao Wang M, M Mengzhen Qiu, M Xinghua Gao, and M Longyang Zhang, Testicular ischemia secondary to acute epididymitis. 2023.

[55]   Hagley M. Epididymo-orchitis and epididymitis: a review of causes and management of unusual forms. Int J STD AIDS 2003; 14(6): 372-8.
[http://dx.doi.org/10.1258/095646203765371240] [PMID: 12816663]

[56]   Fogg RN, Mydlo JH. Nonbacterial infections of the genitourinary tract. Practical Urology: Essential Principles and Practice: Essential Principles and Practice. Springer 2011; pp. 323-37.
[http://dx.doi.org/10.1007/978-1-84882-034-0_24]

[57]   Pathakumari B, Liang G, Liu W. Immune defence to invasive fungal infections: A comprehensive review. Biomed Pharmacother 2020; 130: 110550.
[http://dx.doi.org/10.1016/j.biopha.2020.110550] [PMID: 32739740]

[58]   Nyirjesy P, Sobel JD. Genital mycotic infections in patients with diabetes. Postgrad Med 2013; 125(3): 33-46.
[http://dx.doi.org/10.3810/pgm.2013.05.2650] [PMID: 23748505]

[59]   Naber KG, Bergman B, Bishop MC, *et al.* EAU guidelines for the management of urinary and male genital tract infections. Eur Urol 2001; 40(5): 576-88.
[http://dx.doi.org/10.1159/000049840] [PMID: 11752870]

[60]   Ginindza TG, Stefan CD, Tsoka-Gwegweni JM, *et al.* Prevalence and risk factors associated with sexually transmitted infections (STIs) among women of reproductive age in Swaziland. Infect Agent Cancer 2017; 12(1): 29.
[http://dx.doi.org/10.1186/s13027-017-0140-y] [PMID: 28559923]

[61]   Zhang SJ, Qian HN, Zhao Y, *et al.* Relationship between age and prostate size. Asian J Androl 2013; 15(1): 116-20.
[http://dx.doi.org/10.1038/aja.2012.127] [PMID: 23223031]

[62]   Fenton KA, Korovessis C, Johnson AM, *et al.* Sexual behaviour in Britain: reported sexually transmitted infections and prevalent genital Chlamydia trachomatis infection. Lancet 2001; 358(9296): 1851-4.
[http://dx.doi.org/10.1016/S0140-6736(01)06886-6] [PMID: 11741624]

[63]   Hawkes S, Morison L, Chakraborty J, *et al.* Reproductive tract infections: prevalence and risk factors in rural Bangladesh. Bull World Health Organ 2002; 80(3): 180-8.
[PMID: 11984603]

[64]   Komala M, Kumar KS. Urinary tract infection: causes, symptoms, diagnosis and it's management. Indian Journal of Research in Pharmacy and Biotechnology 2013; 1: 226.

[65]   Svare EI, Kjaer SK, Worm AM, Østerlind A, Meijer CJ, van den Brule AJ. Risk factors for genital HPV DNA in men resemble those found in women: a study of male attendees at a Danish STD clinic. Sex Transm Infect 2002; 78(3): 215-8.
[http://dx.doi.org/10.1136/sti.78.3.215] [PMID: 12238658]

[66]   Okonofua F, Menakaya U, Onemu SO, Omo-Aghoja LO, Bergstrom S. A case-control study of risk factors for male infertility in Nigeria. Asian J Androl 2005; 7(4): 351-61.
[http://dx.doi.org/10.1111/j.1745-7262.2005.00046.x] [PMID: 16281081]

[67]   Sutcliffe S, Giovannucci E, De Marzo AM, Willett WC, Platz EA. Sexually transmitted infections, prostatitis, ejaculation frequency, and the odds of lower urinary tract symptoms. Am J Epidemiol 2005; 162(9): 898-906.
[http://dx.doi.org/10.1093/aje/kwi299] [PMID: 16177142]

[68]   Verze P, Cai T, Lorenzetti S. The role of the prostate in male fertility, health and disease. Nat Rev Urol 2016; 13(7): 379-86.
[http://dx.doi.org/10.1038/nrurol.2016.89] [PMID: 27245504]

[69]   Langan RC. Benign prostatic hyperplasia. Prim Care 2019; 46(2): 223-32.
[http://dx.doi.org/10.1016/j.pop.2019.02.003] [PMID: 31030823]

[70]   Dohle GR. Inflammatory-associated obstructions of the male reproductive tract. Andrologia 2003; 35(5): 321-4.
[http://dx.doi.org/10.1111/j.1439-0272.2003.tb00866.x] [PMID: 14535864]

[71]   Purvis K, Christiansen E. Infection in the male reproductive tract. Impact, diagnosis and treatment in relation to male infertility. Int J Androl 1993; 16(1): 1-13.
[http://dx.doi.org/10.1111/j.1365-2605.1993.tb01146.x] [PMID: 8468091]

[72]   Rivero MJ, Kulkarni N, Thirumavalavan N, Ramasamy R. Evaluation and management of male genital tract infections in the setting of male infertility: an updated review. Curr Opin Urol 2023; 33(3): 180-6.
[http://dx.doi.org/10.1097/MOU.0000000000001081] [PMID: 36861760]

[73]   Gaydos CA. Nucleic acid amplification tests for gonorrhea and chlamydia: practice and applications. Infect Dis Clin North Am 2005; 19(2): 367-386, ix.
[http://dx.doi.org/10.1016/j.idc.2005.03.006] [PMID: 15963877]

[74]   Sharma R, Gupta S, Agarwal A, *et al.* Relevance of leukocytospermia and semen culture and its true place in diagnosing and treating male infertility. World J Mens Health 2022; 40(2): 191-207.
[http://dx.doi.org/10.5534/wjmh.210063] [PMID: 34169683]

[75]   Sindhwani P, Wilson CM. Prostatitis and serum prostate-specific antigen. Curr Urol Rep 2005; 6(4): 307-12.
[http://dx.doi.org/10.1007/s11934-005-0029-y] [PMID: 15978235]

[76]   Grabe M, Bishop M, Bjerklund-Johansen T, Botto H, Çek M, Lobel B, *et al.* Management of urinary and male genital tract infections. Update 2008; 5: 47-60.

[77]   Izuka E, Menuba I, Sengupta P, Dutta S, Nwagha U. Antioxidants, anti-inflammatory drugs and antibiotics in the treatment of reproductive tract infections and their association with male infertility. Chemical Biology Letters 2020; 7: 156-65.

[78]   Gupta R, Wald A, Krantz E, *et al.* Valacyclovir and acyclovir for suppression of shedding of herpes simplex virus in the genital tract. J Infect Dis 2004; 190(8): 1374-81.
[http://dx.doi.org/10.1086/424519] [PMID: 15378428]

[79]   Mendling W, Atef El Shazly M, Zhang L. Clotrimazole for vulvovaginal candidosis: more than 45 years of clinical experience. Pharmaceuticals (Basel) 2020; 13(10): 274.
[http://dx.doi.org/10.3390/ph13100274] [PMID: 32992877]

[80]   Clancy CS, Van Wettere AJ, Siddharthan V, Morrey JD, Julander JG. Comparative histopathologic lesions of the male reproductive tract during acute Infection of Zika virus in AG129 and IFNAR−/− mice. Am J Pathol 2018; 188(4): 904-15.
[http://dx.doi.org/10.1016/j.ajpath.2017.12.019] [PMID: 29378173]

[81]   Muneer A, Macrae B, Krishnamoorthy S, Zumla A. Urogenital tuberculosis — epidemiology, pathogenesis and clinical features. Nat Rev Urol 2019; 16(10): 573-98.
[http://dx.doi.org/10.1038/s41585-019-0228-9] [PMID: 31548730]

[82]   Workowski K A, L H Bachmann, P A Chan, C M Johnston, C A Muzny, I Park, *et al.,* Sexually Transmitted Infections Treatment Guidelines, 2021. MMWR. Recommendations and reports : Morbidity and mortality weekly report. Recommendations and reports. 2021; 70:1-187.

[83]   Sahay S, Deshpande S, Bembalkar S, *et al.* Failure to Use and Sustain Male Condom Usage: Lessons Learned from a Prospective Study among Men Attending STI Clinic in Pune, India. PLoS One 2015; 10(8): e0135071.
[http://dx.doi.org/10.1371/journal.pone.0135071] [PMID: 26270464]

[84]   Gottlieb SL, Low N, Newman LM, Bolan G, Kamb M, Broutet N. Toward global prevention of sexually transmitted infections (STIs): The need for STI vaccines. Vaccine 2014; 32(14): 1527-35.
[http://dx.doi.org/10.1016/j.vaccine.2013.07.087] [PMID: 24581979]

CHAPTER 7

Bacterial Infections and Male Fertility

Abstract: Bacterial infections in the male reproductive system, such as prostatitis, epididymitis, orchitis, urethritis, and balanitis, represent critical health issues contributing to male infertility. Pathogenic microbes infiltrate these reproductive tissues, inciting an immune response, which manifests as inflammation. This immune response is crucial for eradication of the bacterial infestation but can inadvertently inflict collateral damage to the male reproductive tract. Chronic or recurrent inflammation can adversely impact sperm production and function, culminating in a lower sperm count, reduced sperm motility, and abnormal sperm morphology. Furthermore, these infections can lead to erectile dysfunction, amplifying infertility issues. Accurate diagnosis and targeted treatment of these bacterial infections are paramount to mitigate their detrimental effects on male fertility. While bacterial infections are often under-recognized as a cause of male infertility, their impacts are significant and require comprehensive scientific investigation to improve male reproductive health. This chapter underscores the intricate relationship between bacterial infections, the immune response, inflammation, and their effects on male fertility, which aids a basis for innovative therapeutic strategies.

Keywords: Antibiotics, Bacterial Infections, Balanitis, Chlamydia Infections, Epididymitis, *Escherichia coli* Infections, Erectile Dysfunction, Male Infertility, Mycoplasma Infections, Orchitis, Oxidative Stress, Prostatitis, Reproductive Tract Infections, Semen Analysis, Sexually Transmitted Diseases, Sperm Count, Sperm Motility, Spermatozoa, Testis, Urethritis.

INTRODUCTION

Bacterial infections are a significant cause of illness and disease worldwide. Bacterial infections can occur in various parts of the body, including the respiratory system, urinary tract, gastrointestinal tract, and reproductive system. The severity of bacterial infections can range from mild to life-threatening, depending on the type of bacteria involved and the affected body system.

Bacterial infections in the urogenital tract represent significant contributory factors to male infertility [1], with inflammatory conditions and autoimmune complications largely attributed to orchitis, epididymitis, sperm antibody production, or specific immune responses, accounting for approximately 5%–10%

of the causal explanations for male infertility [2, 3]. Among these pathogens, sexually transmitted bacteria such as *Mycoplasma genitalium, Mycoplasma hominis, Ureaplasma urealyticum,* and *Ureaplasma parvum* are notable [4]. *M. genitalium* and *M. hominis* can colonize the urogenital tract, leading to chronic inflammation and immune responses that impair spermatogenesis and sperm function [4, 5]. *M. genitalium* is particularly associated with urethritis, which can progress to epididymitis and orchitis, causing scarring and obstruction of spermatic ducts and the production of antisperm antibodies [5, 6]. *M. hominis,* often found with other infections, can cause epididymitis and prostatitis, affecting sperm quality [7]. Similarly, *U. urealyticum* and *U. parvum,* though part of the normal genital flora, can become pathogenic, leading to conditions like non-gonococcal urethritis, prostatitis, and epididymitis, which negatively impact sperm quality through oxidative stress and inflammation [7, 8]. Understanding these mechanisms is vital for developing effective diagnostic and therapeutic strategies to mitigate the impact of these infections on male reproductive health.

Emerging evidence indicates that inflammation or infection of the genital tract significantly adds to the proportion of idiopathic male infertility cases [9]. Nevertheless, ambiguities persist in the clinical diagnosis and treatment of male urogenital inflammation/infection, primarily due to a lack of comprehensive understanding of the mechanisms underpinning infection-induced male infertility. As bacterial species rank among the most prevalent testicular pathogens, a detailed comprehension of the principal bacterial species causing testicular infections, their virulence factors, and the ensuing immune response is crucial for elucidating the pathophysiology of bacterial-induced male reproductive disturbances. Consequently, this chapter aims to shed light on the most common bacterial infections in the testes, the underlying immune mechanisms, and their impact on male fertility.

BACTERIAL INFECTIONS AND MALE REPRODUCTIVE SYSTEM

Prostatitis

Prostatitis is a term used to describe inflammation of the prostate gland [10]. This condition affects men of all ages, and it is one of the most common urological conditions [10]. Prostatitis can be classified into four different types: acute bacterial prostatitis, chronic bacterial prostatitis, chronic prostatitis/chronic pelvic pain syndrome (CP/CPPS), and asymptomatic inflammatory prostatitis [11].

Acute Bacterial Prostatitis: Acute bacterial prostatitis is a bacterial infection of the prostate gland that usually occurs in younger men [12]. The most common bacteria that cause this type of prostatitis are *Escherichia coli, Klebsiella,* and

Proteus species [13]. Other less common causes include sexually transmitted infections (STIs) such as gonorrhea and chlamydia [13].

Symptoms of acute bacterial prostatitis include sudden onset of fever, chills, urinary urgency, frequency, and pain. Men may also experience pain in the lower back, groin, and perineum (the area between the scrotum and anus). Some men may also experience difficulty starting or stopping urine flow [14].

Diagnosis of acute bacterial prostatitis is made by a combination of symptoms, a physical exam, and laboratory tests. A digital rectal exam (DRE) is often performed to assess the size and consistency of the prostate gland. Urine and blood tests are also performed to confirm the presence of a bacterial infection [14].

Treatment for acute bacterial prostatitis typically involves a course of antibiotics for 2-4 weeks. Pain relief medication and alpha-blockers may also be prescribed to relieve symptoms. In some cases, hospitalization may be necessary for men with severe symptoms [14].

Chronic Bacterial Prostatitis: Chronic bacterial prostatitis is a less common form of prostatitis that is characterized by recurrent bacterial infections of the prostate gland [15]. This type of prostatitis is most common in older men with urinary tract abnormalities, such as an enlarged prostate or urinary catheterization [15].

Symptoms of chronic bacterial prostatitis are similar to those of acute bacterial prostatitis but are often less severe. Men may experience urinary frequency, urgency, and pain during urination. Some men may also experience pain during ejaculation [16].

Diagnosis of chronic bacterial prostatitis is made by a combination of symptoms, a physical exam, and laboratory tests. A DRE is often performed to assess the size and consistency of the prostate gland. Urine and semen cultures are also performed to confirm the presence of a bacterial infection [15].

Treatment for chronic bacterial prostatitis typically involves a longer course of antibiotics, ranging from 4-12 weeks. Pain relief medication and alpha-blockers may also be prescribed to relieve symptoms. In some cases, surgical intervention may be necessary to remove any obstructions in the urinary tract that may be contributing to the infection [17].

Chronic Prostatitis/Chronic Pelvic Pain Syndrome (CP/CPPS): CP/CPPS is the most common type of prostatitis, accounting for approximately 90% of cases. It is a chronic condition characterized by pain and discomfort in the pelvic area that can last for more than three months. The exact cause of CP/CPPS is unknown, but it is believed to be a result of a combination of factors, including inflammation, muscle tension, and nerve damage. Symptoms of CP/CPPS may vary from person to person, but the most common symptoms include pain or discomfort in the pelvic area, lower back, or rectum, pain or burning during urination, frequent urination, especially at night, difficulty starting or stopping urination, painful ejaculation or sexual dysfunction, blood in the urine or semen [18].

Diagnosis of CP/CPPS can be challenging because there is no specific test to diagnose the condition. The diagnosis is usually made based on a combination of symptoms, physical examination, and exclusion of other possible causes of pelvic pain, such as urinary tract infection, prostate cancer, or bladder cancer [18].

Treatment of CP/CPPS aims to relieve symptoms and improve the quality of life of patients [19]. The treatment may include: (a) Antibiotics: Antibiotics may be prescribed if there is evidence of a bacterial infection in the prostate gland; (b) Alpha-blockers: These drugs can help relax the muscles in the prostate and bladder neck, which can reduce the symptoms of urinary frequency and urgency; (c) Pain relievers: Non-steroidal anti-inflammatory drugs (NSAIDs) or other pain relievers may be prescribed to reduce pain and discomfort; (d) Physical therapy: Pelvic floor physical therapy can help reduce muscle tension and improve bladder function; (e) Counseling: Counseling or psychotherapy may be recommended to help patients cope with the emotional and psychological impact of the condition [19].

Asymptomatic Inflammatory Prostatitis: Asymptomatic inflammatory prostatitis is a type of prostatitis that is characterized by inflammation of the prostate gland but no symptoms. It is usually diagnosed incidentally during routine prostate cancer screening or evaluation for other conditions, such as infertility. The exact cause of asymptomatic inflammatory prostatitis is unknown, but it is believed to be a result of an autoimmune or inflammatory response to a viral or bacterial infection. Unlike other types of prostatitis, asymptomatic inflammatory prostatitis does not cause any symptoms, and most patients do not require any treatment [20].

Diagnosis of asymptomatic inflammatory prostatitis is usually made based on the presence of inflammation in the prostate gland, as detected by a prostate biopsy or through other imaging studies. However, it is important to note that the presence of inflammation in the prostate gland does not necessarily indicate the presence of prostate cancer [21].

Treatment of asymptomatic inflammatory prostatitis is usually not necessary unless there is evidence of a bacterial infection, in which case antibiotics may be prescribed. In some cases, close monitoring may be recommended to ensure that the condition does not progress to a more severe form of prostatitis [21].

Epididymitis

Epididymitis is the inflammation of the epididymis, a coiled tube that lies along the posterior surface of the testis and serves as a storage and maturation site for sperm. It is a common condition affecting men of all ages, although it is most common in men between the ages of 19 and 35 [22]. The inflammation may occur unilaterally or bilaterally and may be acute or chronic. It is usually caused by bacterial infection, but other factors such as trauma, chemical exposure, or viral infections may also be implicated [22].

Epididymitis is a prevalent medical phenomenon, with occurrence rates oscillating between 25 to 65 incidents per 10,000 person-years [23]. It is most common in sexually active men between the ages of 19 and 35, although it can occur in men of any age. The condition is more common in men who have sex with men, as well as in men who engage in unprotected sexual activity. In addition, men who have had a history of urinary tract infections or STIs are at a higher risk of developing epididymitis [23].

The most common cause of epididymitis is a bacterial infection, which may occur in the urethra or bladder. The most common bacteria implicated in the development of epididymitis are *Escherichia coli, Klebsiella,* and *Pseudomonas.* Other bacteria, such as *Chlamydia trachomatis* and *Neisseria gonorrhoeae,* may also cause epididymitis, particularly in sexually active men [23]. In addition to bacterial infections, viral infections such as mumps may also cause epididymitis, although this is rare [24]. The inflammation in epididymitis is caused by the activation of the innate immune system in response to the presence of pathogens or other inciting factors. This leads to the release of cytokines, chemokines, and other inflammatory mediators, which cause dilation of blood vessels and an influx of white blood cells into the affected tissue. This results in redness, swelling, pain, and tenderness in the epididymis [23].

The presentation of epididymitis can vary depending on the cause of the condition. In general, patients with epididymitis will present with pain, swelling, and tenderness in the scrotum. The pain may be gradual or sudden in onset and may be accompanied by fever, chills, and nausea [25]. In some cases, patients may also experience dysuria, frequency, or urgency of urination, particularly if the infection has spread to the bladder or urethra. On physical examination, the epididymis is typically tender, swollen, and indurated. In acute cases, the scrotum may be erythematous and edematous. In chronic cases, the epididymis may be palpable as a hard, nodular mass. In some cases, the testis may also be involved, resulting in orchitis [26].

Orchitis

Orchitis is the inflammation of one or both testicles, which are the male reproductive glands responsible for producing and storing sperm. Orchitis can be caused by a bacterial or viral infection, or it can be a result of an injury to the testicles. Inflammation of the testicles can be extremely painful and can lead to long-term complications if left untreated [25].

Orchitis is most commonly caused by a viral infection, specifically the mumps virus [27]. Mumps is a highly contagious viral infection that is spread through respiratory droplets [27]. The virus enters the body through the nose or mouth and then travels to the salivary glands, where it causes inflammation. The virus can also travel to other parts of the body, including the testicles, where it can cause orchitis. Other viruses that can cause orchitis include *Coxsackie virus*, *echovirus*, and HIV [3, 28].

Bacterial infections can also cause orchitis, although this is much less common. Bacteria can enter the testicles through the bloodstream, through a urinary tract infection, or through an STI. STIs that can cause orchitis include *chlamydia* and *gonorrhea* [29]. Rarely, orchitis can be caused by an autoimmune reaction or as a side effect of medication [30].

The most common symptoms of orchitis are pain and swelling in one or both testicles. The pain can be severe and can spread to the groin, abdomen, or lower back. The affected testicle may also feel tender to the touch, and the skin of the scrotum may be warm and red. Other symptoms of orchitis may include fever, chills, headache, nausea, vomiting, and pain during urination. In severe cases, orchitis can lead to complications such as testicular atrophy, abscess formation, or infertility [31].

Urethritis

Urethritis is an inflammation of the urethra, the narrow tube that carries urine from the bladder out of the body. As per data from the Centers for Disease Control and Prevention, there is an annual projection of 19 million novel instances, with approximately 50% observed among the demographic aged 15-24 years [32]. In the context of male urethritis, the microorganisms implicated exhibit the following prevalence rates: *Chlamydia trachomatis* at 33.7%, *Neisseria gonorrhoeae* at 17%, species of *Mycoplasma* at 12%, and species of *Ureaplasma* at 5% [33].

Urethritis can be caused by a variety of factors. The most common cause is a bacterial infection, which is typically sexually transmitted. Non-sexually transmitted bacterial infections can also cause urethritis, such as those caused by *Escherichia coli* and *Klebsiella pneumonia* [34]. Viral infections, such as herpes simplex virus, can also cause urethritis. In addition to infections, urethritis can also be caused by chemical irritants, such as soaps, lotions, and perfumes [35]. Some people may be sensitive to certain chemicals, which can cause irritation and inflammation of the urethra. Other causes of urethritis include trauma to the urethra, such as from catheterization or sexual activity, and an enlarged prostate gland, which can cause a blockage of the urethra [36].

The symptoms of urethritis can vary depending on the cause of the inflammation. However, common symptoms of urethritis include pain or discomfort during urination, a frequent urge to urinate, and a discharge from the penis or vagina. Men may also experience pain or swelling in the testicles or penis, and women may experience pain in the lower abdomen or during sexual intercourse [37].

Balanitis

Balanitis refers to the inflammatory condition of the penile glans, also known as the apex of the penis. This condition is characterized by inflammation of the foreskin and the head of the penis, which can lead to itching, pain, discharge, and redness. Balanitis can be caused by a variety of factors, including poor hygiene, skin allergies, fungal or bacterial infections, and sexually transmitted diseases [38].

This pathology is relatively prevalent, with an estimated lifetime incidence among the male population ranging between 3 to 11 percent [39]. The incidence of balanitis is higher in uncircumcised males, particularly in those who do not maintain good genital hygiene.

There are various causes of balanitis, and they can be broadly classified into infectious and non-infectious causes. The infectious causes of balanitis include bacterial, fungal, and viral infections. Bacterial infections can be caused by a variety of organisms, including *Streptococcus, Staphylococcus*, and *E. coli*. Fungal infections, particularly candidiasis, are also a common cause of balanitis [40]. Viral infections such as herpes simplex virus can also lead to balanitis. Non-infectious causes of balanitis include poor hygiene, skin allergies, and dermatological conditions such as psoriasis and lichen planus. Other factors that can contribute to balanitis include the use of irritant soaps or detergents, tight-fitting clothing, and exposure to certain chemicals [40].

The symptoms of balanitis can vary depending on the underlying cause. However, common symptoms include redness, itching, pain, and discharge from the penis. In some cases, there may be an unpleasant odor or a rash on the penis. If left untreated, balanitis can lead to more severe symptoms, such as ulceration, scarring, and difficulty retracting the foreskin [38].

The best way to prevent balanitis is to maintain good genital hygiene. This includes washing the penis and foreskin daily with mild soap and water and drying the area thoroughly. Uncircumcised males should also retract the foreskin during washing to remove any debris or smegma that may accumulate. Using condoms during sexual intercourse can also help prevent the transmission of STIs that can lead to balanitis [38].

IMMUNE MECHANISM OF BACTERIAL INFESTATION IN MALE REPRODUCTIVE TRACT

The testes demonstrate several innate immune responses, particularly*via*Toll-Like Receptor (TLR) activated pathways [41]. These are instigated by bacterial factors binding to various TLRs on testicular cells, causing receptor dimerization and intracellular signaling, eventually activating transcription factors such as nuclear factor-κB (NFκB) and mitogen-activated protein kinases (MAPKs), including extracellular signal-regulated kinase (ERK), p38, and c-Jun N-terminal kinase (JNK) [42, 43] Fig. (**9**).

Five adaptor molecules help facilitate this process, one of which, the myeloid differentiation primary-response protein 88 (MyD88), is key, while TLR3 and TLR4 employ the TIR-domain containing adaptor protein inducing IFNβ (TRIF) [44]. TLRs expressed in testes include TLRs-2,3,4, and 9, with TLR-2 and 4 recognizing diacyl lipoproteins or gram-positive bacteria and Lipopolysaccharide ligands or gram-negative bacteria respectively [45, 46].

Signaling pathways related to TLR-4 result in the rapid activation of NF-κβ and subsequent production of inflammatory cytokines, or alternatively activate Interferon Regulatory Factor– 3 (IRF3), instigating the transcription of interferon-α/β (IFN-α/β), and interferon γ induced protein (IP)-10 [47, 48]. TLR signaling also facilitates antigen-presenting cell maturation and adaptive immune responses [49].

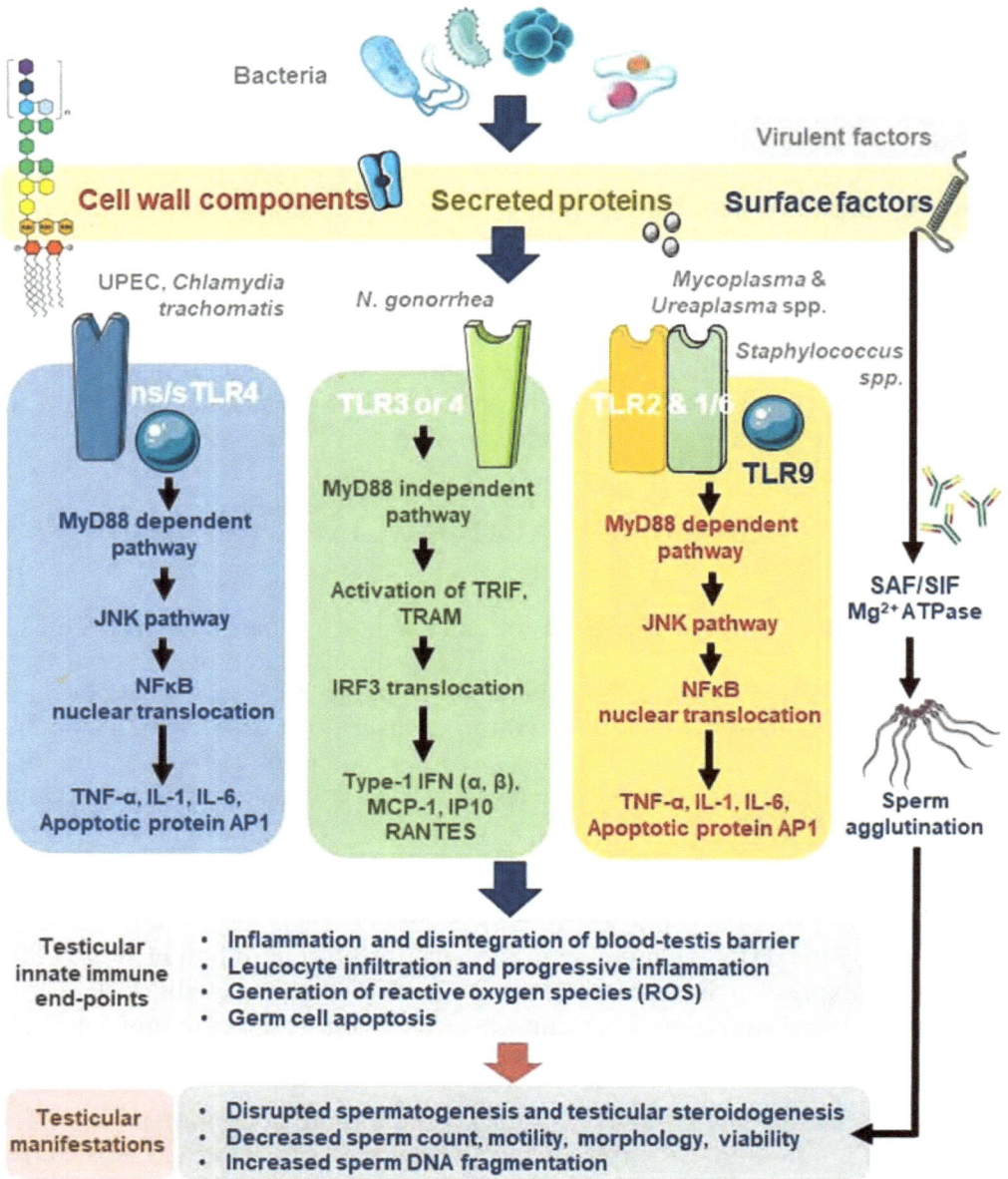

Fig. (9). Bacterial infection-mediated testicular innate immune pathways and their impact on testicular functions.

However, bacterial virulence factors can subvert these immune responses, inhibiting NF κβ signaling, thus reducing inflammatory responses [50, 51]. For instance, Uropathogenic Escherichia coli (UPEC) and non-pathogenic E. coli

(NPEC) can suppress the release of proinflammatory responses even when activating the MyD88-dependent TLR4 signaling pathway, possibly due to NF κβ suppression [50, 51].

Furthermore, bacterial Lipopolysaccharides (LPS) can activate TLR3 signaling, triggering anti-viral responses*via*MyD88-independent pathways. These pathways involve TRIF and TRIF-related adapter molecule (TRAM), leading to the phosphorylation of interferon-regulated factor (IRF)-3 in the infected testicular cells, which then induces apoptotic and antiviral responses [52, 53]. This subversion of pro-inflammatory signaling by bacterial ligands allows bacteria to survive within the testes, providing insight into how bacteria modulate proinflammatory cytokine secretion at various phases of testicular innate immune signaling Fig. (**9**).

EFFECTS OF BACTERIAL INFECTIONS ON MALE FERTILITY

Bacterial infections can have a significant impact on male fertility. The male reproductive system is vulnerable to various infections, including bacterial infections, which can cause a range of problems that affect the quantity, quality, and movement of sperm. In this chapter, we will explore the effects of bacterial infections on male fertility [54, 55].

Lower Sperm Count

Bacterial infections in the male reproductive system can cause inflammation that damages the testes and lowers the production of sperm. Infections can also interfere with the transport of sperm, leading to lower sperm count. For example, epididymitis, a bacterial infection of the epididymis, which is a coiled tube located behind each testicle, can cause lower sperm count [56]. This infection can cause inflammation that narrows or blocks the epididymis, making it difficult for sperm to move through the tube. Similarly, orchitis, which is a bacterial infection of the testicles, can also lead to lower sperm count. This infection can cause swelling and inflammation in the testicles, which can damage the cells that produce sperm, leading to a reduction in sperm count [57].

Reduced Sperm Motility

Bacterial infections can also affect the ability of sperm to move properly. Sperm motility is essential for fertilization, and any damage to the sperm or its environment can affect its ability to move toward the egg. Bacterial infections can cause inflammation that damages the lining of the epididymis and testicles, leading to a buildup of white blood cells and other fluids that can hinder the movement of sperm. Additionally, infections can lead to the production of antibodies that attack and damage the sperm, reducing their motility [56].

Abnormal Sperm Morphology

Bacterial infections can damage the testicles, epididymis, or other structures in the male reproductive system, leading to changes in sperm morphology [58]. One example of a bacterial infection that affects sperm morphology is *Chlamydia trachomatis* [59]. This STI can cause inflammation of the epididymis, leading to scarring and blockage of the ducts that transport sperm from the testicles. This can result in abnormal sperm morphology, including reduced sperm count, motility, and viability. *E. coli* is another bacterium that enters the urinary tract or prostate gland and causes infections affecting sperm morphology. *E. coli* infection can lead to inflammation of the prostate gland, which can damage the gland's cells and ducts. This can result in decreased sperm count, motility, and abnormal morphology [60].

Gonorrhea, another STI, can also affect sperm morphology. Gonorrhea can cause inflammation of the urethra, prostate gland, and epididymis, leading to the formation of scar tissue [61]. This can cause blockage of the ducts that transport sperm, resulting in abnormal sperm morphology and reduced sperm count. In addition to STIs, bacterial infections that affect the general health of the body can also impact sperm morphology [61]. For example, infections that cause high fever can affect sperm morphology by raising the body's temperature above the normal range. This can impair sperm production, leading to reduced sperm count and abnormal morphology. Bacterial infections can also indirectly affect sperm morphology by causing inflammation throughout the body. Inflammation triggers the production of free radicals, which can damage cells, including sperm cells. Free radicals can damage the DNA of the sperm, leading to abnormal morphology and reduced fertility [56, 62].

Thus, bacterial infections can significantly impact male fertility by affecting sperm morphology. Infections such as *Chlamydia trachomatis, Escherichia coli,* and *Gonorrhea* can cause inflammation and scarring in the male reproductive system, leading to reduced sperm count, motility, and viability. Other infections that cause high fever or inflammation throughout the body can indirectly affect sperm morphology by producing free radicals that damage sperm cells. Early diagnosis and treatment of bacterial infections can prevent or minimize the damage they cause to the male reproductive system and improve the chances of a successful pregnancy.

Erectile Dysfunction

Bacterial infections can directly or indirectly affect male fertility by interfering with the normal physiological processes that regulate the male reproductive system [55, 56, 58]. One of the most common bacterial infections associated with erectile dysfunction (ED) is *Chlamydia trachomatis*, which is a sexually transmitted bacterium that can cause urethritis, epididymitis, and prostatitis [63]. *Chlamydia trachomatis* infections can cause ED by inducing an inflammatory response that damages the endothelium of the penile blood vessels. This can result in reduced blood flow to the penis, making it difficult to achieve or maintain an erection. In addition, Chlamydia trachomatis infections can lead to the formation of scar tissue in the penis, which can further impair erectile function. Another bacterial infection that can cause ED is prostatitis, which is an inflammation of the prostate gland. Prostatitis can be caused by a variety of bacterial pathogens, including *E coli* and *Klebsiella pneumoniae*. The inflammation associated with prostatitis can damage the nerves and blood vessels that regulate erectile function, leading to ED [64].

Bacterial infections can also indirectly contribute to ED by causing systemic inflammation [65]. Inflammatory cytokines such as interleukin-1 (IL-1), interleukin-6 (IL-6), and tumor necrosis factor-alpha (TNF-α) are produced in response to bacterial infections and can interfere with the normal physiological processes that regulate erectile function. For example, these cytokines can impair the production of nitric oxide (NO), a molecule that is essential for the normal function of the penile blood vessels. In addition to bacterial infections, other risk factors for ED include obesity, smoking, alcohol consumption, and certain medications. These risk factors can interact with bacterial infections to exacerbate the development of ED [65].

Thus, bacterial infections can contribute to the development of ED by directly damaging the penile blood vessels or indirectly by causing systemic inflammation. Chlamydia trachomatis and prostatitis are two bacterial infections that are commonly associated with ED. Treatment of these infections typically involves antibiotics and lifestyle modifications. Early diagnosis and treatment of bacterial infections can help prevent the development of ED and improve overall male fertility [66].

CONCLUSION

Bacterial infections in the male reproductive system represent a substantial yet under-researched factor contributing to male infertility. Chronic inflammation caused by persistent bacterial infection can lead to anatomical and functional alterations within the male reproductive tract. Prostatitis, or inflammation of the prostate, often induced by bacterial infection, can cause discomfort and potential fertility issues. Epididymitis, inflammation of the epididymis frequently resulting from bacterial infection, can disrupt normal sperm maturation. Orchitis, bacterial infection-driven inflammation of the testicles, can negatively impact sperm production and testosterone secretion. Urethritis, primarily bacterial in origin, can lead to painful urination and potential fertility complications. Balanitis, inflammation of the glans penis often resulting from bacterial infection, can cause pain, erectile dysfunction, and potentially impair fertility.

Bacterial infections trigger a complex immune response in the male reproductive system involving innate and adaptive immunity, which can result in inflammation and tissue damage. Bacterial infections in the male reproductive system can lead to a lower sperm count, reducing the chances of successful fertilization. They can affect sperm motility, thus diminishing the ability of sperm to reach and fertilize an egg, and can also induce abnormal sperm morphology, impairing the sperm's fertilizing capacity. Persistent bacterial infections can cause erectile dysfunction, posing an additional barrier to natural conception. Cumulative effects of bacterial infections in the male reproductive system can result in infertility.

The impact of bacterial infections on male fertility is substantial, necessitating more research to better understand the underlying mechanisms, improve diagnostic methods, and develop more effective treatment strategies.

REFERENCES

[1]   Henkel R, Solomon M. Semen culture and the assessment of genitourinary tract infections. Indian J Urol 2017; 33(3): 188-93.
[http://dx.doi.org/10.4103/iju.IJU_407_16] [PMID: 28717267]

[2]   Dohle G, Colpi G, Hargreave T, Papp G, Jungwirth A, Weidner W. EAU guidelines on male infertility. Eur Urol 2005; 48(5): 703-11.
[http://dx.doi.org/10.1016/j.eururo.2005.06.002] [PMID: 16005562]

[3]   Schuppe HC, Meinhardt A, Allam JP, Bergmann M, Weidner W, Haidl G. Chronic orchitis: a neglected cause of male infertility? Andrologia 2008; 40(2): 84-91.
[http://dx.doi.org/10.1111/j.1439-0272.2008.00837.x] [PMID: 18336456]

[4]   Alzaidi JR, Kareem AA. The Impact of Urogenital Tract Infectious Bacteria on Male Fertility. Medical Journal of Babylon 2024; 21(2): 476-80.
[http://dx.doi.org/10.4103/MJBL.MJBL_75_24]

[5]   Sarier M, Kukul E. Classification of non-gonococcal urethritis: a review. Int Urol Nephrol 2019; 51(6): 901-7.
[http://dx.doi.org/10.1007/s11255-019-02140-2] [PMID: 30953260]

[6]   Taylor-Robinson D, Horner PJ. The role of Mycoplasma genitalium in non-gonococcal urethritis. The Medical Society for the Study of Venereal Disease 2001; pp. 229-31.

[7]   Cheng C, Chen X, Song Y, *et al.* Genital mycoplasma infection: a systematic review and meta-analysis. Reprod Health 2023; 20(1): 136.
[http://dx.doi.org/10.1186/s12978-023-01684-y] [PMID: 37700294]

[8]   Zuber A, Peric A, Pluchino N, Baud D, Stojanov M. Human male genital tract microbiota. Int J Mol Sci 2023; 24(8): 6939.
[http://dx.doi.org/10.3390/ijms24086939] [PMID: 37108103]

[9]   Schuppe H-C, Meinhardt A. Immune privilege and inflammation of the testis. Immunology of Gametes and Embryo Implantation. Karger Publishers 2005; pp. 1-14.
[http://dx.doi.org/10.1159/000087816]

[10]   Magri V, Boltri M, Cai T, *et al.* Multidisciplinary approach to prostatitis. Arch Ital Urol Androl 2019; 90(4): 227-48.
[http://dx.doi.org/10.4081/aiua.2018.4.227] [PMID: 30655633]

[11]   Weidner W, Anderson RU. Evaluation of acute and chronic bacterial prostatitis and diagnostic management of chronic prostatitis/chronic pelvic pain syndrome with special reference to infection/inflammation. Int J Antimicrob Agents 2008; 31 (Suppl. 1): 91-5.
[http://dx.doi.org/10.1016/j.ijantimicag.2007.07.044] [PMID: 18162376]

[12]   Beland L, Martin C, Han JS. Lower urinary tract symptoms in young men—causes and management. Curr Urol Rep 2022; 23(2): 29-37.
[http://dx.doi.org/10.1007/s11934-022-01087-9] [PMID: 35132519]

[13]   Škerk V, Schönwald S, Krhen I, *et al.* Aetiology of chronic prostatitis. Int J Antimicrob Agents 2002; 19(6): 471-4.
[http://dx.doi.org/10.1016/S0924-8579(02)00087-0] [PMID: 12135835]

[14]   Coker TJ, Dierfeldt DM. Acute bacterial prostatitis: diagnosis and management. Am Fam Physician 2016; 93(2): 114-20.
[PMID: 26926407]

[15]   Su ZT, Zenilman JM, Sfanos KS, Herati AS. Management of chronic bacterial prostatitis. Curr Urol Rep 2020; 21(7): 29.
[http://dx.doi.org/10.1007/s11934-020-00978-z] [PMID: 32488742]

[16]   Rees J, Abrahams M, Doble A, Cooper A, Group PER. Diagnosis and treatment of chronic bacterial prostatitis and chronic prostatitis/chronic pelvic pain syndrome: a consensus guideline. BJU Int 2015; 116(4): 509-25.
[http://dx.doi.org/10.1111/bju.13101] [PMID: 25711488]

[17]   Khamdamov B, Yodgorov I. Assessment of the effectiveness of diagnosis and therapy of patients with chronic bacterial prostatitis. Sci Prog 2022; 3: 31-3.

[18]   Zhang J, Liang C, Shang X, Li H. Chronic prostatitis/chronic pelvic pain syndrome: a disease or symptom? Current perspectives on diagnosis, treatment, and prognosis. Am J Men Health 2020; 14(1)
[http://dx.doi.org/10.1177/1557988320903200] [PMID: 32005088]

[19]   Magistro G, Wagenlehner FME, Grabe M, Weidner W, Stief CG, Nickel JC. Contemporary management of chronic prostatitis/chronic pelvic pain syndrome. Eur Urol 2016; 69(2): 286-97.
[http://dx.doi.org/10.1016/j.eururo.2015.08.061] [PMID: 26411805]

[20]   Taoka R, Kakehi Y. The influence of asymptomatic inflammatory prostatitis on the onset and progression of lower urinary tract symptoms in men with histologic benign prostatic hyperplasia. Asian J Urol 2017; 4(3): 158-63.
[http://dx.doi.org/10.1016/j.ajur.2017.02.004] [PMID: 29264225]

[21]   Videčnik Zorman J, Matičič M, Jeverica S, Smrkolj T. Diagnosis and treatment of bacterial prostatitis. Acta Dermatovenerol Alp Panonica Adriat 2015; 24(2): 25-9.
[PMID: 26086164]

[22]   Meinhardt A, Michel V, Pilatz A, Hedger MP. Epididymitis: revelations at the convergence of clinical and basic sciences. Asian J Androl 2015; 17(5): 756-63.
[http://dx.doi.org/10.4103/1008-682X.155770] [PMID: 26112484]

[23] Çek M, Sturdza L, Pilatz A. Acute and chronic epididymitis. Eur Urol Suppl 2017; 16(4): 124-31.
[http://dx.doi.org/10.1016/j.eursup.2017.01.003]

[24] Roychoudhury S, Das A, Sengupta P, *et al.* Viral pandemics of twenty-first century. J Microbiol Biotechnol Food Sci 2021; 10(4): 711-6.
[http://dx.doi.org/10.15414/jmbfs.2021.10.4.711-716]

[25] Pain A S, Prostatitis, Epididymitis, and Orchitis. Introduction to Clinical Infectious Diseases: A Problem-Based Approach. 2019.

[26] Khastgir J. Advances in the antibiotic management of epididymitis. Expert Opin Pharmacother 2022; 23(9): 1103-13.
[http://dx.doi.org/10.1080/14656566.2022.2062228] [PMID: 35380486]

[27] Wu H, Wang F, Tang D, Han D. Mumps orchitis: clinical aspects and mechanisms. Front Immunol 2021; 12: 582946.
[http://dx.doi.org/10.3389/fimmu.2021.582946] [PMID: 33815357]

[28] Akhigbe RE, Dutta S, Hamed MA, Ajayi AF, Sengupta P, Ahmad G. Viral infections and male infertility: a comprehensive review of the role of oxidative stress. Frontiers in Reproductive Health 2022; 4: 782915.
[http://dx.doi.org/10.3389/frph.2022.782915] [PMID: 36303638]

[29] Monleon R, Martin MP, John Barnes H. Bacterial orchitis and epididymo-orchitis in broiler breeders. Avian Pathol 2008; 37(6): 613-7.
[http://dx.doi.org/10.1080/03079450802499134] [PMID: 19023758]

[30] Pannek J, Haupt G. Orchitis due to vasculitis in autoimmune diseases. Scand J Rheumatol 1997; 26(3): 151-4.
[http://dx.doi.org/10.3109/03009749709065674] [PMID: 9225868]

[31] Azmat C E and P Vaitla, Orchitis. 2020.

[32] Samra Z, Rosenberg S, Madar-Shapiro L. Direct simultaneous detection of 6 sexually transmitted pathogens from clinical specimens by multiplex polymerase chain reaction and auto-capillary electrophoresis. Diagn Microbiol Infect Dis 2011; 70(1): 17-21.
[http://dx.doi.org/10.1016/j.diagmicrobio.2010.12.001] [PMID: 21392925]

[33] Khatib N, Bradbury C, Chalker V, *et al.* Prevalence of *Trichomonas vaginalis*, *Mycoplasma genitalium* and *Ureaplasma urealyticum* in men with urethritis attending an urban sexual health clinic. Int J STD AIDS 2015; 26(6): 388-92.
[http://dx.doi.org/10.1177/0956462414539464] [PMID: 24925897]

[34] Woolley PD, Kinghorn GR, Talbot MD, Duerden BI. Microbiological flora in men with non-gonococcal urethritis with particular reference to anaerobic bacteria. Int J STD AIDS 1990; 1(2): 122-5.
[http://dx.doi.org/10.1177/095646249000100210] [PMID: 2092786]

[35] Berntsson M, Löwhagen G-B, Bergström T, *et al.* Viral and bacterial aetiologies of male urethritis: findings of a high prevalence of Epstein–Barr virus. Int J STD AIDS 2010; 21(3): 191-4.
[http://dx.doi.org/10.1258/ijsa.2009.009262] [PMID: 20215624]

[36] Bachmann LH, Manhart LE, Martin DH, *et al.* Advances in the understanding and treatment of male urethritis. Clin Infect Dis 2015; 61 (Suppl. 8): S763-9.
[http://dx.doi.org/10.1093/cid/civ755] [PMID: 26602615]

[37] Young A, Toncar A, Wray AA. Urethritis. StatPearls. StatPearls Publishing 2022. Internet

[38] Charlton OA, Smith SD. Balanitis xerotica obliterans: a review of diagnosis and management. Int J Dermatol 2019; 58(7): 777-81.
[http://dx.doi.org/10.1111/ijd.14236] [PMID: 30315576]

[39] Edwards S. Balanitis and balanoposthitis: a review. Genitourin Med 1996; 72(3): 155-9.

[PMID: 8707315]

[40]   Wray AA, Velasquez J, Khetarpal S. Balanitis. StatPearls. StatPearls Publishing 2022. Internet

[41]   Dutta S, Sengupta P, Hassan MF, Biswas A. Role of toll-like receptors in the reproductive tract inflammation and male infertility. Chemical Biology Letters 2020; 7: 113-23.

[42]   Oshiumi H, Matsumoto M, Funami K, Akazawa T, Seya T. TICAM-1, an adaptor molecule that participates in Toll-like receptor 3–mediated interferon-β induction. Nat Immunol 2003; 4(2): 161-7.
[http://dx.doi.org/10.1038/ni886] [PMID: 12539043]

[43]   Yamamoto M, Sato S, Hemmi H, *et al.* TRAM is specifically involved in the Toll-like receptor 4–mediated MyD88-independent signaling pathway. Nat Immunol 2003; 4(11): 1144-50.
[http://dx.doi.org/10.1038/ni986] [PMID: 14556004]

[44]   Carty M, Goodbody R, Schröder M, Stack J, Moynagh PN, Bowie AG. The human adaptor SARM negatively regulates adaptor protein TRIF–dependent Toll-like receptor signaling. Nat Immunol 2006; 7(10): 1074-81.
[http://dx.doi.org/10.1038/ni1382] [PMID: 16964262]

[45]   Nishimura M, Naito S. Tissue-specific mRNA expression profiles of human toll-like receptors and related genes. Biol Pharm Bull 2005; 28(5): 886-92.
[http://dx.doi.org/10.1248/bpb.28.886] [PMID: 15863899]

[46]   Riccioli A, Starace D, Galli R, *et al.* Sertoli cells initiate testicular innate immune responses through TLR activation. J Immunol 2006; 177(10): 7122-30.
[http://dx.doi.org/10.4049/jimmunol.177.10.7122] [PMID: 17082629]

[47]   Bhushan S, Schuppe HC, Tchatalbachev S, *et al.* Testicular innate immune defense against bacteria. Mol Cell Endocrinol 2009; 306(1-2): 37-44.
[http://dx.doi.org/10.1016/j.mce.2008.10.017] [PMID: 19010387]

[48]   Girling JE, Hedger MP. Toll-like receptors in the gonads and reproductive tract: emerging roles in reproductive physiology and pathology. Immunol Cell Biol 2007; 85(6): 481-9.
[http://dx.doi.org/10.1038/sj.icb.7100086] [PMID: 17592495]

[49]   Iwasaki A, Medzhitov R. Toll-like receptor control of the adaptive immune responses. Nat Immunol 2004; 5(10): 987-95.
[http://dx.doi.org/10.1038/ni1112] [PMID: 15454922]

[50]   Bhushan S, Hossain H, Lu Y, *et al.* Uropathogenic E. coli induce different immune response in testicular and peritoneal macrophages: implications for testicular immune privilege. PLoS One 2011; 6(12): e28452.
[http://dx.doi.org/10.1371/journal.pone.0028452] [PMID: 22164293]

[51]   Ruckdeschel K, Mannel O, Richter K, *et al.* Yersinia outer protein P of Yersinia enterocolitica simultaneously blocks the nuclear factor-κ B pathway and exploits lipopolysaccharide signaling to trigger apoptosis in macrophages. J Immunol 2001; 166(3): 1823-31.
[http://dx.doi.org/10.4049/jimmunol.166.3.1823] [PMID: 11160229]

[52]   Di Pietro M, Filardo S, Alfano V, *et al. Chlamydia trachomatis* elicits TLR3 expression but disrupts the inflammatory signaling down-modulating NFκB and IRF3 transcription factors in human Sertoli cells. J Biol Regul Homeost Agents 2020; 34(3): 977-86.
[PMID: 32664712]

[53]   O'Neill LAJ, Bowie AG. The family of five: TIR-domain-containing adaptors in Toll-like receptor signalling. Nat Rev Immunol 2007; 7(5): 353-64.
[http://dx.doi.org/10.1038/nri2079] [PMID: 17457343]

[54]   Oghbaei H, Rastgar Rezaei Y, Nikanfar S, *et al.* Effects of bacteria on male fertility: Spermatogenesis and sperm function. Life Sci 2020; 256: 117891.
[http://dx.doi.org/10.1016/j.lfs.2020.117891] [PMID: 32504760]

[55]   Dutta S, Sengupta P, Izuka E, Menuba I, Jegasothy R, Nwagha U. Staphylococcal infections and infertility: mechanisms and management. Mol Cell Biochem 2020; 474(1-2): 57-72.
[http://dx.doi.org/10.1007/s11010-020-03833-4] [PMID: 32691256]

[56]   Sanocka-Maciejewska D, Ciupińska M, Kurpisz M. Bacterial infection and semen quality. J Reprod Immunol 2005; 67(1-2): 51-6.
[http://dx.doi.org/10.1016/j.jri.2005.06.003] [PMID: 16112738]

[57]   Zeyad A, Hamad MF, Hammadeh ME. The effects of bacterial infection on human sperm nuclear protamine P1/P2 ratio and DNA integrity. Andrologia 2018; 50(2): e12841.
[http://dx.doi.org/10.1111/and.12841] [PMID: 28736810]

[58]   Zeyad A, Amor H, Eid Hammadeh M. The impact of bacterial infections on human spermatozoa. Int J Women's Health Reprod Sci 2017; 5(4): 243-52.
[http://dx.doi.org/10.15296/ijwhr.2017.43]

[59]   Moazenchi M, Totonchi M, Salman Yazdi R, *et al.* The impact of *Chlamydia trachomatis* infection on sperm parameters and male fertility: A comprehensive study. Int J STD AIDS 2018; 29(5): 466-73.
[http://dx.doi.org/10.1177/0956462417735245] [PMID: 29065772]

[60]   Diemer T, Huwe P, Michelmann HW, Mayer F, Schiefer HG, Weidner W. *Escherichia coli* -induced alterations of human spermatozoa. An electron microscopy analysis. Int J Androl 2000; 23(3): 178-86.
[http://dx.doi.org/10.1046/j.1365-2605.2000.00224.x] [PMID: 10844544]

[61]   Umapathy E. STD/HIV association: effects on semen characteristics. Arch Androl 2005; 51(5): 361-5.
[http://dx.doi.org/10.1080/014850190924124] [PMID: 16087564]

[62]   Dutta S, Sengupta P, Slama P, Roychoudhury S. Oxidative stress, testicular inflammatory pathways, and male reproduction. Int J Mol Sci 2021; 22(18): 10043.
[http://dx.doi.org/10.3390/ijms221810043] [PMID: 34576205]

[63]   Uts S. R f, O Ziganshin, Y M Raigorodsky, and E Sultanakhmedov, The role of combined physiotherapy in the treatment of the persistent forms of Chlamydial prostatitis complicated by erectile dysfunction. Russian Journal of Physiotherapy. Balneology and Rehabilitation 2015; 14: 30-7.

[64]   Clark C. Erectile dysfunction and other problems: clinical. S Afr Pharm J 2008; 75: 32-6.

[65]   Kaya-Sezginer E, Gur S. The inflammation network in the pathogenesis of erectile dysfunction: attractive potential therapeutic targets. Curr Pharm Des 2020; 26(32): 3955-72.
[http://dx.doi.org/10.2174/1381612826666200424161018] [PMID: 32329680]

[66]   Manfredi C, Castiglione F, Fode M, Lew-Starowicz M, Romero-Otero J, Bettocchi C, *et al.* News and future perspectives of non-surgical treatments for erectile dysfunction. Int J Impot Res 2022; 1-7.
[PMID: 35896717]

CHAPTER 8

Paradigm of Viral Infections and Dynamics in the Male Reproductive System

Abstract: The interaction between viral infections and male reproductive health has significant implications for fertility and warrants a comprehensive understanding. This chapter examines the complex mechanisms through which viruses, including sexually transmitted viruses such as Human Immunodeficiency Virus (HIV), Human Papillomavirus (HPV), Herpes Simplex Virus (HSV), and emerging infections such as Severe Acute Respiratory Syndrome Coronavirus 2 (SARS-CoV-2), can invade and impact the male reproductive system. Attention is particularly given to the consequences of these infections on aspects of male fertility, including the quantification and evaluation of sperm count, morphology, and motility. Further, the chapter explores the dual role of the immune response within the male reproductive system during viral infections, elucidating the delicate balance between immunoprotection and immunopathology. Moreover, it offers an in-depth analysis of existing and potential therapeutic strategies, with a focus on antiviral medications, vaccination approaches, and immune modulation techniques. Thus, this chapter aims to provide a comprehensive understanding of the dynamics of viral infections in the male reproductive system to facilitate the development of effective countermeasures against these infections.

Keywords: Epididymitis, Hepatitis Virus, Herpes Genitalis, HIV Infections, Human Papillomavirus Infection, Male Urogenital Diseases, Orchitis, Prostatitis, Reproduction, Reproductive Tract Infections, Seminal Vesiculitis, Spermatozoa, Testicular Diseases, Testis, Urethritis, Urogenital Neoplasms, Urogenital System, Urologic Diseases, Viral Load, Virus Replication.

INTRODUCTION

Viral infections pose a significant healthcare challenge to humans, as their ramifications extend beyond the initial acute stage of infection. Notably, a plethora of viral infections have been implicated in a variety of long-term health detriments, inclusive of complications in the sphere of reproductive health [1].

Viruses inciting these infections can be partitioned into four primary categories contingent upon their genetic composition: DNA viruses, RNA viruses, retroviruses, and pararetroviruses. Such infections, commonly reported in humans, comprise influenza, human papillomavirus (HPV), herpes simplex virus (HSV), human immunodeficiency virus (HIV), hepatitis B virus (HBV), and hepatitis C virus (HCV) [1].

Apart from their immediate health repercussions, these infections notably hold substantial implications for male reproductive health. They have been correlated with a range of conditions, such as infertility, erectile dysfunction, prostate anomalies, sexually transmitted infections (STIs), and testicular cancer [2]. Mitigation of the adverse effects of viral infections on male reproductive health is primarily reliant on prevention. Comprehensive strategies involve immunization, adoption of safe sexual conduct, rigorous adherence to hygiene protocols, and prompt treatment of existing viral infections; these measures collectively serve to diminish the likelihood of enduring complications [2]. In this chapter, we aim to present a concise summary of viral infections, underscoring their relationship with and influence on male reproductive health.

VIRAL INFECTIONS AFFECTING THE MALE REPRODUCTIVE SYSTEM

Viruses are one of the most common causes of infections in humans, and they can infect various organs and tissues of the body, including the male reproductive system [3, 4] Fig. (**10**).

Human Papillomavirus (HPV)

HPV is a sexually transmitted virus that can cause a wide range of health problems, including cancers of the cervix, anus, penis, vulva, and oropharynx [5]. While HPV is commonly associated with cervical cancer in women [6], it is also a significant health concern for men, as it can affect their reproductive system [7].

HPV is a highly prevalent virus, with an estimated 79 million Americans currently infected with some type of HPV [8]. While there are more than 100 types of HPV, about 40 types can infect the genital area [9]. HPV is typically spread through sexual contact, including vaginal, anal, and oral sex. Most people who contract HPV do not experience any symptoms and clear the virus on their own within a few years. However, in some cases, HPV can persist and cause health problems, including genital warts and cancer [9]. Genital warts are a common symptom of HPV in both men and women. In men, genital warts can appear on the penis, scrotum, or around the anus [10, 11]. Warts may be single or multiple and can vary in size and shape. While genital warts themselves are not cancerous, they can be uncomfortable and may cause social and psychological distress. Treatment options for genital warts include topical medications, cryotherapy (freezing), laser therapy, or surgical removal [10, 12]. In addition to causing genital warts, HPV is also a risk factor for penile cancer. While penile cancer is relatively rare, accounting for less than 1% of all cancers in men, it can be a serious and potentially life-threatening condition [13]. Research has shown that HPV infection is associated with about half of all cases of penile cancer. In particular, HPV types 16 and 18 are most commonly associated with penile cancer [14]. Other risk factors for penile cancer include smoking, poor hygiene, and a history of phimosis (a condition in which the foreskin cannot be retracted). Symptoms of penile cancer may include a growth or sore on the penis, bleeding, or discharge. Treatment options for penile cancer depend on the stage and severity of the cancer, and may include surgery, radiation therapy, and chemotherapy [14].

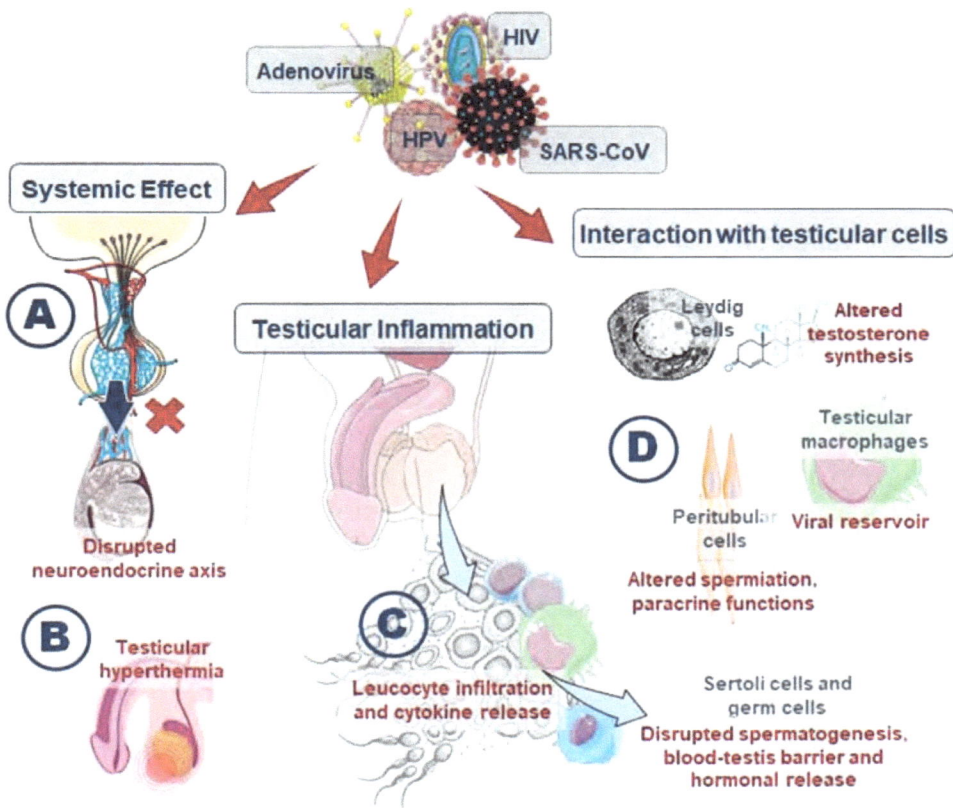

Fig. (10). Viral infections induced male reproductive disruption. A. Viral infections may cause systemic dyshomeostasis impairing endocrine regulation of reproductive functions; B. Viral infections-induced testicular hyperthermia leads to spermatogenic impairments; C. Viruses may invade testes directly inflicting testicular inflammation; D. Viral infections and inflammation may disrupt testicular immune homeostasis. Testicular somatic cells like Leydig cells and Sertoli cells interact with the activated immune cells, thereby affecting normal testicular functions.

While HPV is not typically associated with severe male infertility, there is some evidence to suggest that it may have an impact on sperm quality and fertility [15]. Research has shown that men with HPV may have a higher incidence of abnormal sperm morphology (shape) and reduced sperm motility (movement) [15, 16]. Additionally, some studies have found that HPV DNA can be present in semen samples from infected men, which may increase the risk of transmitting the virus to sexual partners [17]. However, the clinical significance of HPV in semen samples and its impact on fertility is still being studied, and more research is needed to fully understand the relationship between HPV and male fertility. The most effective way to prevent HPV infection and the associated health problems is through vaccination [18]. The HPV vaccine is recommended for both boys and girls starting at age 11 or 12 and can be administered up to age 26 [19, 20]. The vaccine is most effective when given before sexual activity begins, as it cannot prevent infection with HPV types that a person has already been exposed to. In addition to vaccination, practicing safe sex can help reduce the risk of HPV and other sexually transmitted infections. This includes using condoms and limiting the number of sexual partners [18].

Herpes Simplex Virus (HSV)

HSV is a common virus that can cause a range of infections, including genital herpes [21, 22]. While genital herpes can affect both men and women, it is particularly important to understand the implications of the virus for male reproductive health. In this chapter, we will explore the ways in which HSV can impact male reproductive health, including its effects on fertility and the transmission of the virus to sexual partners [23, 24]. Herpes simplex virus is a DNA virus that can cause a variety of clinical manifestations, including cold sores (oral herpes) and genital herpes. Genital herpes is caused by two types of the virus: HSV-1 and HSV-2. Both types can cause genital herpes, but HSV-2 is the most common cause of genital herpes [21, 22].

The most common symptoms of genital herpes in men include sores or blisters on the penis or around the genital area, itching, burning, and pain during urination [25]. These symptoms typically appear within two weeks after infection and can be accompanied by flu-like symptoms such as fever, headaches, and body aches. One of the major concerns for men with genital herpes is the impact of the virus on their reproductive health. While genital herpes does not typically cause long-term health problems, it can affect male fertility in a number of ways [23]. First, genital herpes can lead to inflammation in the reproductive organs, including the testicles and prostate gland. This inflammation can interfere with the production and quality of sperm, potentially leading to reduced fertility. In addition, HSV can cause damage to the DNA of sperm cells, which can impact the ability of these cells to fertilize an egg. This damage can also increase the risk of birth defects in any offspring that are conceived through the affected sperm [26]. Finally, genital herpes can lead to psychological stress and anxiety, which can also impact male fertility. The stress associated with the diagnosis and management of genital herpes can cause hormonal imbalances that interfere with the production of sperm [27]. It is important to note that while genital herpes can impact male fertility, the virus does not typically cause permanent infertility. In many cases, the effects on fertility are temporary and can be reversed with appropriate treatment [28]. In addition to the impact on male fertility, genital herpes can also impact the transmission of the virus to sexual partners. Men with genital herpes can transmit the virus to their partners through sexual contact, even when they do not have any visible symptoms [29]. In fact, the majority of genital herpes infections are transmitted by individuals who are asymptomatic or who have very mild symptoms that are not recognized as herpes. This makes the virus difficult to control, as individuals may be unaware that they are infected and are, therefore, more likely to transmit the virus to others [29].

To reduce the risk of transmission, it is important for men with genital herpes to use barrier methods such as condoms during sexual activity and to avoid sexual contact during outbreaks of the virus. Men with genital herpes should also communicate openly with their sexual partners about their diagnosis and the risks of transmission. In addition to these measures, antiviral medications can be used to manage the symptoms of genital herpes and reduce the risk of transmission [30]. These medications, such as acyclovir, valacyclovir, and famciclovir, work by inhibiting the replication of the virus, reducing the severity and duration of outbreaks. In conclusion, herpes simplex virus is a common infection that can have a range of impacts on male reproductive health [23]. While the virus can cause inflammation, damage to DNA, and psychological stress that can impact male fertility, the effects are typically temporary and can be managed with appropriate treatment. In addition, men with genital herpes can reduce the risk of transmission to sexual partners through the use of barrier methods and antiviral medications, as well as open communication about the risks of transmission.

Human Immunodeficiency Virus (HIV)

HIV is a virus that attacks the immune system of the human body, leading to an increased risk of infections and diseases [31]. HIV is primarily transmitted through sexual contact, sharing needles or syringes, and mother-to-child transmission during pregnancy, childbirth, or breastfeeding [31]. While HIV affects both males and females, there are specific concerns related to male reproductive health that need to be addressed [2, 4].

HIV infection has several implications for male reproductive health. It can impact fertility, sexual function, and the development of reproductive organs. HIV can also increase the risk of certain conditions such as testicular cancer, prostate cancer, and other STIs [32, 33]. HIV can impact fertility by causing damage to the male reproductive organs. Research has shown that HIV can cause damage to the testicles, leading to a reduction in sperm count, motility, and morphology. These changes in sperm parameters can impact the ability to achieve a successful pregnancy. Additionally, HIV-positive men may have a lower sex drive, leading to reduced sexual activity and lower chances of conception [34, 35]. HIV can impact sexual function in several ways. Erectile dysfunction, premature ejaculation, and decreased libido are commonly reported in HIV-positive men [36]. These symptoms may be related to HIV infection itself or the side effects of antiretroviral therapy. It is a treatment used to manage HIV, and certain medications used in antiretroviral therapy have been associated with sexual dysfunctions [37]. Additionally, HIV-positive men may experience sexual dysfunction due to psychological stress and anxiety related to their HIV status. HIV can also impact the development of reproductive organs in males [38]. Studies have shown that HIV-positive men may experience a delay in the onset of puberty, leading to delayed development of the testicles and penis [39]. This delay in puberty can result in reduced sperm production and lower levels of testosterone, impacting sexual function and fertility [40].

HIV-positive men have a higher risk of developing testicular cancer than HIV-negative men [41]. Research has shown that the risk of testicular cancer is increased in men with a weakened immune system, such as those with HIV [42]. Testicular cancer is a rare but serious form of cancer that requires prompt diagnosis and treatment. Studies have shown that HIV-positive men may have a higher risk of developing prostate cancer than HIV-negative men. This risk is thought to be related to the increased risk of certain STIs, such as HPV and hepatitis B and C, which are known to be risk factors for prostate cancer [43]. HIV-positive men are at increased risk of contracting other STIs, such as gonorrhea, chlamydia, and syphilis. These infections can lead to further complications, such as infertility, if left untreated. Additionally, certain STIs, such as herpes and HPV, have been associated with an increased risk of certain types of cancer, including cervical, anal, and penile cancers [44]. While HIV can have a significant impact on male reproductive health, there are various strategies that can be used to manage these issues. Some of the approaches are discussed here.

Antiretroviral therapy is the primary treatment for HIV, which employs a mix of medications that suppress the virus and inhibit its replication, contributing to reducing the viral load, improving male reproductive health, and potentially preventing HIV transmission to sexual partners [45]. Hormone replacement therapy (HRT) helps manage hormonal imbalances brought on by HIV and ART by supplementing or replacing the natural hormonal milieu of the body, improving libido, reducing erectile dysfunction, and boosting overall sexual functionality [46]. Erectile dysfunction medications, including sildenafil (Viagra), tadalafil (Cialis), and vardenafil (Levitra), are used to treat erectile dysfunction induced by HIV and ART, working by enhancing blood flow to the penis, consequently improving erections [47]. Fertility treatments such as *in vitro* fertilization (IVF) and intracytoplasmic sperm injection (ICSI) assist men with HIV and infertility in conceiving; these processes involve sperm retrieval, egg fertilization in a lab, and then embryo transfer to the woman's uterus [48].

Coronavirus

Since the 2002 SARS-CoV pandemic, research indicates possible coronavirus invasion into human reproductive systems [49], transmitted*via*inhalation or contact with infected individuals [50]. The virus utilizes angiotensin-converting enzyme 2 (ACE2) receptors for cellular entry, initiating a replication and inflammatory process involving p38 mitogen-activated protein kinases (MAPK) and extracellular-regulated protein kinases (ERK) [51, 52].

Regarding reproduction, it is postulated that SARS-CoV-2 might trigger MAPK/ERK signaling, with males exhibiting a higher ACE2 receptor density [53, 54]. Sperm cells, Leydig cells, and Sertoli cells manifest significant ACE2 expression, yet evidence of viral presence in male semen is inconsistent [54]. Hypothetically, compromised blood-testis barriers during inflammation could allow viral invasion [55, 56]. COVID-19 patients reportedly exhibit increased serum luteinizing hormone (LH) and reduced serum testosterone levels [57], suggesting a direct viral impact on testicular tissues, potentially through oxidative-sensitive MAPK/ERK-mediated hyper-inflammatory pathways [58].

Indirect effects encompass germ cell destruction and testicular dysfunction from temperature elevations, as well as Leydig cell hyperplasia in some cases [55]. Infected individuals might exhibit disrupted Leydig cell functionality, reduced testosterone production, and a compromised blood-testis barrier [53].

Previous coronaviruses, notably SARS-CoV, have been associated with orchitis and potential spermatogenesis disruption [53]. IgG deposition in testicular tissues has been observed, hinting at inflammation-mediated testicular damage and oxidative stress (OS) generation. Psychological stress, an OS trigger, is correlated with depression and post-traumatic stress disorder [59], though the exact link remains unclear. SARS-CoV-2, like SARS-CoV, is thought to evade stress responses, potentially increasing organ inflammation [60]. At a cellular level, oxidative damage can result in membrane lipid peroxidation and sperm DNA fragmentation, impairing spermatogenesis and leading to male infertility [61].

DYNAMICS OF VIRAL INFECTIONS IN THE MALE REPRODUCTIVE SYSTEM

Understanding How Viruses Enter and Interact with the Male Reproductive System

The entry of viruses into the male reproductive system can have serious consequences, including infertility and reduced sexual function [62]. It is important to explore the dynamics of viral infections in the male reproductive system, focusing on how viruses enter and interact with the organs of the male reproductive system. Understanding how viruses enter the male reproductive system is essential to understanding how they cause infections. The male reproductive system is protected by a physical barrier that prevents pathogens from entering the system. However, certain viruses can bypass this barrier and enter the reproductive system through different pathways [63].

HPV and HSV are sexually transmitted viruses that can enter the male reproductive system through the urethra during sexual intercourse. Once inside the male reproductive system, HPV and HSV can infect the epithelial cells of the urethra and cause inflammation and sores [62]. CMV and HIV can also enter the male reproductive system through the bloodstream. CMV can infect the testes and cause inflammation and reduced sperm production [64]. HIV can also infect the testes and cause inflammation, leading to reduced sperm quality and quantity. Zika virus can infect the male reproductive system. It is primarily transmitted through the bite of infected mosquitoes, but it can also be transmitted sexually. Once inside the male reproductive system, the Zika virus can infect the testes and cause inflammation and reduced sperm production. The mechanisms of viral entry into the male reproductive system are complex and require further study to fully understand [65].

Once inside the male reproductive system, viruses can interact with different organs and tissues in different ways. Understanding how viruses interact with the male reproductive system is essential to developing effective treatment strategies [3, 64]. When a virus infects the male reproductive system, the immune system of the body responds by releasing cytokines and other inflammatory molecules. This immune response can lead to inflammation and damage to the male reproductive system [66].

Viruses instigate an inflammatory response that leads to conditions such as urethritis (urethral inflammation), prostatitis (prostatic inflammation), epididymitis (epididymal inflammation), and orchitis (testicular inflammation). These pathogens prompt the activation of the host's innate immune system, which results in leukocyte invasion and an elevation of proinflammatory cytokines [4, 64]. While such inflammation facilitates the innate capacity of the organism to counter viral incursions, it may also stimulate the production of reactive oxygen species (ROS) and disturb the redox equilibrium, causing subsequent oxidative damage [3, 66]. This places reproductive structures, particularly the urethra, prostate, and epididymis, at risk for inflammatory and oxidative harm. Furthermore, epididymal sperm cells, along with spermatozoa in transit during ejaculation, become susceptible to the detrimental impacts of cytokines and ROS. These factors contribute to a decline in sperm count, a reduction in sperm motility, and a decrease in the number of sperm cells exhibiting normal morphology [56, 66].

Cytokines, interleukin (IL)-1, IL-1, 6, and tumor necrosis factor (TNF)-α regulate testicular functions based on environmental factors [63]. In normal states, they ensure homeostasis of the blood-testis barrier and foster immune protection of the testis, thereby supporting healthy spermatogenesis [63]. Conversely, proinflammatory cytokine overexpression triggers blood-testis barrier restructuring through Cldn 11 deregulation in Sertoli cells and induces germ cell apoptosis*via*activation of TNFR1, IL-6R, and FAS [67]. Furthermore, cytokines compromise male fertility by impeding sperm motility, inhibiting testosterone production*via*TLR-2 and TLR-4 activation on spermatozoa membranes, and mediating a self-perpetuating cycle of OS*via*ROS induction [66].

Increased OS predisposes testes and spermatozoa plasma membranes, rich in polyunsaturated fatty acid (PUFA), to ROS-mediated oxidation, resulting in lipid peroxidation, compromised cell membrane integrity, and elevated ion permeability [68]. Subsequent oxidative damage to the nuclear chromatin leads to DNA base modifications and fragmentation, culminating in testicular and sperm cell apoptosis [68]. As a result, viral infections may directly alter semen quality, damage DNA integrity, and produce anti-sperm antibodies, disrupting steroidogenesis, sperm motility, and sperm-oocyte binding, thus impairing fertilization*via*inflammation and OS pathways [66].

Interestingly, certain antiviral drugs, effective against viruses, have been shown to affect male fertility. For example, ribavirin damages germ cells*via*cell growth inhibition, causing apoptosis, and Interferon (IFN) α-2b, effective against mumps, may induce oligoasthenozoospermia [69, 70]. Steroids suppress testosterone production, and various antivirals effective against HIV may impair testicular and sperm function. Such treatments can induce seminiferous tubule atrophy and disrupt spermatogenesis, reduce testosterone levels due to Leydig cell mass reduction, and cause testicular and sperm cell DNA fragmentation, erectile dysfunction, and reduced fertility indices [71].

Explanation of Viral Persistence and Latency

One important concept in the study of viral infections is viral persistence. This refers to the ability of a virus to establish a long-term infection in a host, even in the presence of a functioning immune system. Viral persistence can be caused by a variety of factors, including the ability of the virus to hide from the immune system, the ability to establish a reservoir of infected cells, or the ability to integrate its genetic material into the host genome [62]. In the male reproductive system, viral persistence can have significant impacts on fertility and reproductive health. Another important concept in the study of viral infections is viral latency. This refers to the ability of a virus to remain dormant in a host for extended periods of time without causing any symptoms or actively replicating [65]. Viral latency can be caused by a variety of factors, including the ability of the virus to establish a stable reservoir in the host, the ability to suppress the host's immune response, or the ability to switch between active replication and latency. In the male reproductive system, viral latency can be particularly problematic because it can make it difficult to diagnose and treat infections [65]. For example, HSV can establish a latent infection in the ganglia that supply the genitals, which can reactivate periodically and cause painful genital sores. These outbreaks can be treated with antiviral medications, but they do not cure the underlying infection. In some cases, HSV can also cause a chronic, low-level infection that is difficult to diagnose and treat [72].

The immunological regulation in the testes accomplishes two critical functions: it shields the germ cells that express auto-antigens from systemic immune responses and simultaneously facilitates a selective innate immune defense against invading pathogens [73]. The testicular microenvironment, characterized by immune privilege and suppression, fosters the tolerance of allo- and auto-antigens without prompting immune rejection [74, 75]. Consequently, this renders the testes a possible sanctuary for viruses, permitting them to survive for extended periods, ranging from several months to years [76, 77].

The concept of testicular immune privilege was initially postulated by John Hunter in 1767, deduced from the transplantation of a cock's testis into a hen's abdominal cavity and later recovering it in a morphologically altered state [78]. During the 1910s-1930s, numerous experimental testicular transplants were conducted among humans and in laboratory settings [78]. Notably, when ovaries were transplanted into the testes, the latter was found to safeguard the development of ovarian follicles over several months [79]. Subsequent research in the 1970s-1980s further revealed that different types of xenografts and allografts could persist functionally in the testes for a considerable period [80]. Particularly, the testes tolerated 'insulin-secreting xenogeneic islets' for a substantially longer period compared to other recipient sites [81].

The immune system, through its development, learns to tolerate self-antigens. However, germ cells in the testes start expressing auto-antigens during puberty, a phase when systemic immune competence is already established. The immune system perceives these germ cell auto-antigens as foreign entities [82]. Hence, the testes' tolerogenic property is crucial to prevent potentially harmful immune responses, thereby shielding auto-antigenic germ cells by obscuring them from the systemic immune system [83]. The downside to testicular tolerance and immune privilege is that certain harmful viruses may find refuge in these organs [76, 84]. Viruses may persist in the testes even after the individual has recovered from the infection, potentially leading to secondary viral transmission through sexual activity [85 - 87].

Viruses residing in the testes can induce latent viral infections, which occur when the infected cell harbors the dormant, non-replicating virus [85, 88]. Such a latent virus maintains its entire viral genome, and upon cessation of latency, it can resume replication, producing infectious viruses and causing re-infection. The latent virus can also integrate into the host human genome or persist in the host cell nucleus as an episome, a self-replicating piece of DNA [89, 90]. The recurrence of infection by the reactivated latent virus in the testis can occur several months or even years after the initial infection [62, 91].

Initially, it was believed that the absence of lymphatic drainage in the testes contributed to their immune privilege. However, this theory was refuted with the discovery of afferent lymphatic vessels in the testes [82]. It was then hypothesized that the blood-testis barrier (BTB) was responsible for isolating the auto-antige--bearing germ cells from the immune system, thereby conferring the testes with immune privilege [92]. Further research revealed that cells in the testicular interstitium and early-stage germ cells (spermatogonia and preleptotene spermatocytes) situated outside the BTB also benefit from this immune privilege [78, 93]. The findings indicate that spermatids and spermatozoa are not shielded from the immune system by the BTB alone, but rather germ cells evade immune rejection through the intricate and finely balanced immune regulation within the testes [78, 94]. This nuanced local immunity in the testis is preserved by the coordinated functions of all testicular cells, including germ cells, Sertoli cells, Leydig cells, peritubular myoid cells, interstitial dendritic cells, macrophages, blood vessel endothelia, and lymphocytes [67, 74, 82].

The dynamics of viral infections in the male reproductive system are complex and multifaceted. In addition to the concepts of viral persistence and latency, there are a number of other factors that can influence the course of these infections, including the host's immune response, the presence of other infections or comorbidities, and the characteristics of the virus itself. For example, HIV infection can have a significant impact on the male reproductive system, both through direct effects on the reproductive organs and through the impact of the virus on the immune system. HIV can infect and replicate in the testes and epididymis, leading to inflammation and damage to the reproductive tissues. This can result in a variety of reproductive health problems, including erectile dysfunction, testicular atrophy, and decreased sperm production [35]. In addition, HIV infection can also cause a range of systemic effects that can impact the male reproductive system. For example, HIV can suppress the immune system, making it more difficult for the body to fight off other infections. This can increase the risk of other sexually transmitted infections, which can further impact fertility and reproductive health [65, 95].

DISCUSSION OF THE POTENTIAL LONG-TERM CONSEQUENCES OF VIRAL INFECTIONS ON REPRODUCTIVE HEALTH

In addition to the immediate impact that viral infections can have on male fertility, there may also be long-term consequences that can impact reproductive health. Some of the potential long-term consequences of viral infections on reproductive health are discussed below.

Increased risk of infertility: One of the most significant long-term consequences of viral infections on male fertility is an increased risk of infertility. This is particularly true for infections that cause inflammation in the testicles or prostate gland, as this can lead to permanent damage to these organs [96, 97].

Increased risk of birth defects: Viral infections can also increase the risk of birth defects in children. This is because some viral infections can cause damage to the DNA of sperm cells, which can lead to genetic abnormalities in offspring [98 - 100].

Increased risk of miscarriage: Viral infections can also increase the risk of miscarriage in women. This is because some viral infections can cause damage to the DNA of sperm cells, which can lead to genetic abnormalities in offspring [101, 102].

Increased risk of cancer: Some viral infections, such as HPV, can increase the risk of certain types of cancer, including testicular cancer. This is because the virus can cause damage to the DNA of cells, which can lead to abnormal growth and division [41].

DIAGNOSIS AND TREATMENT

Methods of Diagnosing Viral Infections in the Male Reproductive System

Viral infections can cause a wide range of symptoms in the male reproductive system, including testicular pain, swelling, and inflammation. The diagnosis of viral infections in the male reproductive system typically involves a combination of medical history, physical examination, and laboratory testing [103].

Medical History

The first step in diagnosing a viral infection in the male reproductive system is to obtain a detailed medical history. The patient will be asked about his symptoms, including the location, duration, and severity of the pain, as well as any other symptoms he may be experiencing, such as fever or rash. The physician will also ask about any recent sexual activity or exposure to other individuals with known viral infections [104].

Physical Examination

After obtaining a medical history, a physical examination of the male reproductive system will be performed. The physician will examine the testicles, scrotum, and penis for any signs of swelling, redness, or inflammation. In some cases, a rectal exam may be performed to assess the prostate gland.

Laboratory Testing

Laboratory testing is an essential component of the diagnostic process for viral infections in the male reproductive system [105]. The following tests may be performed:

Blood tests: Blood tests can detect the presence of viral antibodies or other markers of infection. For example, the presence of HPV antibodies in the blood may indicate an active or past infection with the virus [106].

Urine tests: Urine tests can detect the presence of viral particles in the urine. This type of test is commonly used to diagnose HSV and cytomegalovirus (CMV) infections [107].

Semen analysis: Semen analysis is a test that evaluates the quality and quantity of sperm in a semen sample. In cases of viral infections, the semen sample may be tested for the presence of viral particles [108].

Biopsy: In some cases, a biopsy may be performed to obtain a tissue sample for laboratory analysis. This type of test may be necessary if the physician suspects

the presence of a viral infection that cannot be detected through other diagnostic methods [109].

Approaches to Treating Viral Infections and Associated Symptoms

Treating viral infections can be challenging, as there are no specific antiviral medications available for some of these conditions. However, there are several approaches to treating viral infections in the male reproductive system, including antiviral medications, immunotherapy, and surgery [110].

Antiviral Medications

Antiviral medications are a common treatment for viral infections in the male reproductive system [71]. These medications work by blocking the replication of the virus, preventing it from spreading and causing further damage [105]. One of the most common antiviral medications used to treat viral infections in the male reproductive system is acyclovir. This medication is often used to treat HSV, which can cause painful sores and blisters on the genitals. Acyclovir is typically taken orally and can also be applied topically to the affected area [111]. Another antiviral medication used to treat viral infections in the male reproductive system is ganciclovir. This medication is often used to treat cytomegalovirus, which can cause inflammation of the prostate gland and testicles. Ganciclovir is typically administered intravenously and may also be used in combination with other medications [112].

Immunotherapy

Immunotherapy is another approach to treating viral infections in the male reproductive system. This approach involves using the body's own immune system to fight off the virus by boosting the body's natural defenses and targeting the virus directly [113]. One form of immunotherapy used to treat viral infections in the male and female reproductive system is interferon therapy. Interferons are a type of protein that helps regulate the immune system and can be used to stimulate the natural systemic defenses against viruses [114]. Interferon therapy is often used to treat hepatitis B and C, which can cause inflammation and damage to the liver. Another form of immunotherapy used to treat viral infections in the male reproductive system is therapeutic vaccines. These vaccines are designed to stimulate the immune system to recognize and attack the virus by introducing a weakened or dead form of the virus into the body. Therapeutic vaccines are still in development for many viral infections, including HPV and HIV [115, 116].

Surgery

Surgery is another approach to treating viral infections in the male reproductive system. While not a direct treatment for the virus itself, surgery can be used to remove damaged tissue or repair damage caused by the infection. One form of surgery used to treat viral infections in the male reproductive system is circumcision. Circumcision involves the removal of the foreskin of the penis, which can reduce the risk of infection with certain viruses like HPV and HIV [117]. Circumcision may also be recommended for men who experience recurrent infections or inflammation of the foreskin. Another form of surgery used to treat viral infections in the male reproductive system is testicular biopsy. This procedure involves removing a small sample of tissue from the testicles, which can be examined for signs of infection or damage. Testicular biopsy may be used to diagnose conditions like CMV or other viral infections that can affect the testicles [117, 118].

PREVENTION AND FUTURE RESEARCH

Importance of Prevention and Protective Measures Against Viral Infections

Prevention and protective measures are important in minimizing the impact of viral infections on the male reproductive tract. Some of these measures include:

Safe Sex Practices: One of the most effective ways to prevent viral infections in the male reproductive tract is through safe sex practices. This includes using condoms and practicing monogamy or abstinence [119].

Vaccinations: Vaccinations can help prevent some viral infections, such as HPV. Vaccinations are especially important for young men who are sexually active [120].

Good Hygiene: Good hygiene practices can help prevent the spread of viral infections. This includes washing hands regularly and avoiding contact with bodily fluids [121].

Avoiding High-Risk Behaviors: High-risk behaviors, such as sharing needles, can increase the risk of contracting viral infections [121].

Treatment of Viral Infections: Treating viral infections as soon as possible can help minimize their impact on the male reproductive tract. This includes taking antiviral medications and seeking medical treatment as soon as symptoms appear [121].

Potential Future Research in this Field

As the research horizon expands toward the examination of viral infections in the male reproductive tract, several prospective research trajectories are emerging. Central to these investigations is the elucidation of the distinct interaction dynamics between viral pathogens and the male reproductive system.

Initially, the processes by which viruses enter and persist within the male genital tract have yet to be completely clarified. A more profound understanding of these molecular interactions might provide targets for innovative prophylactic strategies or potentially curative treatments for established infections [65]. In particular, a more extensive exploration of viral exploitation of host cell receptors, alongside triggered immunological responses, could contribute to the design of more effective antiviral therapies.

Furthermore, the role of the microbiome within the male reproductive tract warrants deeper investigation. The interaction dynamics between resident microbiota and viral pathogens have the potential to alter susceptibility to and outcomes of these infections [122]. Thus, microbiome modulation may present a novel approach for preventing and treating viral infections in the male reproductive tract.

Precision medicine also holds considerable potential in future research paradigms. A thorough understanding of individual susceptibility, which may be influenced by genetic, epigenetic, and environmental factors, could facilitate personalized prevention and treatment strategies [123]. Consequently, more exhaustive and diverse genomic studies integrating multi-omics data are crucial for advancing our understanding in this field.

An additional area requiring attention is the long-term effect of viral infections on male fertility [124]. Achieving a comprehensive understanding of how these infections influence sperm quality and function, as well as the possibility for vertical virus transmission during conception, is an essential research objective. These studies gain particular significance in the context of emergent viruses such as Zika and COVID-19, which are known to exert effects on the male reproductive system [2].

Lastly, socio-behavioral dimensions should not be neglected. Increased comprehension of how cultural, educational, and behavioral factors can affect the prevalence and outcome of these infections may significantly improve intervention strategies. More holistic, intersectional studies focusing on these factors could yield invaluable insights.

Thus, the research frontier of viral infections in the male reproductive tract is abundant with opportunities. Progress in technology, coupled with our expanding comprehension of the intricate nature of virus-host interactions, paves the way for innovative, multifaceted research initiatives. The ultimate aim of these collective endeavors is to enhance preventive measures, improve therapeutic options, and protect male reproductive health against the threat of viral infections.

CONCLUSION

Viral infections can significantly affect the male reproductive system, leading to diverse and often severe consequences. The understanding of these infections and their dynamics is essential to safeguard male fertility. Common viruses such as HPV, HSV, HIV, Zika virus, and coronaviruses can have significant impacts on the male reproductive system, leading to conditions like infertility, cancer, and STIs.

The dynamics of viral infections include their invasion, replication, and interaction with the host cells. The balance between host immunity and viral pathogenicity defines the outcomes of these infections. Viruses enter the male reproductive system through various routes, such as sexual transmission, blood-borne transmission, and vertical transmission. Once inside, they interact with host cells, evade the immune response, and establish infection. Some viruses exhibit persistence and latency within the male reproductive system. They can exist in a dormant state for extended periods, evading the host's immune system and causing recurring symptoms or becoming active under certain conditions. Viral infections can negatively impact male fertility by affecting sperm production, causing inflammation and damage to reproductive tissues, and potentially leading to male infertility. This impact is seen across various viruses and is a significant cause for concern. Diagnosing viral infections in the male reproductive system involves a variety of methods, including physical examination, serological tests, polymerase chain reaction (PCR), and imaging techniques. Treatment strategies focus on managing symptoms, reducing viral load, and preventing transmission. Antiviral drugs, immunotherapy, and supportive treatments are commonly used.

Future research aims at further understanding the viral infection dynamics in the male reproductive system, developing better diagnostic tools, and devising more effective treatments. More research is also needed to understand the long-term impacts of viral infections on male fertility and to develop preventive strategies.

REFERENCES

[1] Fields BN. Fields' virology. Lippincott Williams & Wilkins 2007.

[2] Roychoudhury S, Das A, Sengupta P, *et al.* Viral pandemics of the last four decades: pathophysiology, health impacts and perspectives. Int J Environ Res Public Health 2020; 17(24): 9411.
[http://dx.doi.org/10.3390/ijerph17249411] [PMID: 33333995]

[3] Akhigbe RE, Dutta S, Hamed MA, Ajayi AF, Sengupta P, Ahmad G. Viral infections and male infertility: a comprehensive review of the role of oxidative stress. Frontiers in Reproductive Health 2022; 4: 782915.
[http://dx.doi.org/10.3389/frph.2022.782915] [PMID: 36303638]

[4] Roychoudhury S, Das A, Sengupta P, *et al.* Viral pandemics of twenty-first century. J Microbiol Biotechnol Food Sci 2021; 10(4): 711-6.
[http://dx.doi.org/10.15414/jmbfs.2021.10.4.711-716]

[5] Forman D, de Martel C, Lacey CJ, *et al.* Global burden of human papillomavirus and related diseases. Vaccine 2012; 30 (Suppl. 5): F12-23.
[http://dx.doi.org/10.1016/j.vaccine.2012.07.055] [PMID: 23199955]

[6] Okunade KS. Human papillomavirus and cervical cancer. J Obstet Gynaecol 2020; 40(5): 602-8.
[http://dx.doi.org/10.1080/01443615.2019.1634030] [PMID: 31500479]

[7] Goulart ACX, Farnezi HCM, França JPBM, Santos A, Ramos MG, Penna MLF. HIV, HPV and Chlamydia trachomatis: impacts on male fertility. JBRA Assist Reprod 2020; 24(4): 492-7.
[http://dx.doi.org/10.5935/1518-0557.20200020] [PMID: 32496735]

[8] Kovar CL, Pestaner M, Webb Corbett R, Rose CL. HPV vaccine promotion: Snapshot of two health departments during the COVID-19 pandemic. Public Health Nurs 2021; 38(5): 715-9.
[http://dx.doi.org/10.1111/phn.12900] [PMID: 33938032]

[9] Trottier H, Franco EL. The epidemiology of genital human papillomavirus infection. Vaccine 2006; 24 (Suppl. 1): S4-S15.
[http://dx.doi.org/10.1016/j.vaccine.2005.09.054] [PMID: 16406226]

[10] Baer H, Allen S, Braun L. Knowledge of human papillomavirus infection among young adult men and women: implications for health education and research. J Community Health 2000; 25(1): 67-78.
[http://dx.doi.org/10.1023/A:1005192902137] [PMID: 10706210]

[11] Karnes JB, Usatine RP. Management of external genital warts. Am Fam Phys 2014; 90(5): 312-8.
[PMID: 25251091]

[12] Manhart LE, Koutsky LA. Do condoms prevent genital HPV infection, external genital warts, or cervical neoplasia? A meta-analysis. Sex Transmit Dis 2002; pp. 725-35.

[13] Stratton KL, Culkin DJ. A contemporary review of HPV and penile cancer. Oncology (Williston Park) 2016; 30(3): 245-9.
[PMID: 26984219]

[14] Iorga L, Dragos Marcu R, Cristina Diaconu C, *et al.* Penile carcinoma and HPV infection (Review). Exp Ther Med 2020; 20(1): 91-6.
[PMID: 32518604]

[15] Foresta C, Noventa M, De Toni L, Gizzo S, Garolla A. HPV-DNA sperm infection and infertility: from a systematic literature review to a possible clinical management proposal. Andrology 2015; 3(2): 163-73.
[http://dx.doi.org/10.1111/andr.284] [PMID: 25270519]

[16]   Moghimi M, Zabihi-Mahmoodabadi S, Kheirkhah-Vakilabad A, Kargar Z. Significant correlation between high-risk HPV DNA in semen and impairment of sperm quality in infertile men. Int J Fertil Steril 2019; 12(4): 306-9.
        [PMID: 30291691]

[17]   Capra G, Schillaci R, Bosco L, Roccheri MC, Perino A, Ragusa MA. HPV infection in semen: results from a new molecular approach. Epidemiol Infect 2019; 147: e177.
        [http://dx.doi.org/10.1017/S0950268819000621] [PMID: 31063107]

[18]   Zou K, Huang Y, Li Z. Prevention and treatment of human papillomavirus in men benefits both men and women. Front Cell Infect Microbiol 2022; 12: 1077651.
        [http://dx.doi.org/10.3389/fcimb.2022.1077651] [PMID: 36506029]

[19]   Arbyn M, de Sanjosé S, Saraiya M, *et al.* EUROGIN 2011 roadmap on prevention and treatment of HPV-related disease. Int J Cancer 2012; 131(9): 1969-82.
        [http://dx.doi.org/10.1002/ijc.27650] [PMID: 22623137]

[20]   Meites E, Kempe A, Markowitz L. Use of a 2-dose schedule for human papillomavirus vaccination—updated recommendations of the advisory committee on immunization practices. Elsevier 2017; pp. 834-7.

[21]   Ross JD, Smith IW, Elton RA. The epidemiology of herpes simplex types 1 and 2 infection of the genital tract in Edinburgh 1978-1991. Sex Transm Infect 1993; 69(5): 381-3.
        [http://dx.doi.org/10.1136/sti.69.5.381] [PMID: 8244358]

[22]   Lafferty WE, Downey L, Celum C, Wald A. Herpes simplex virus type 1 as a cause of genital herpes: impact on surveillance and prevention. J Infect Dis 2000; 181(4): 1454-7.
        [http://dx.doi.org/10.1086/315395] [PMID: 10762576]

[23]   Seyed H, Mostafa S, Mohammadali K, *et al.* Asymptomatic seminal infection of herpes simplex virus. J Biomed Res 2013; 27(1): 56-61.
        [http://dx.doi.org/10.7555/JBR.27.20110139] [PMID: 23554795]

[24]   Kurscheidt FA, Damke E, Bento JC, *et al.* Effects of herpes simplex virus infections on seminal parameters in male partners of infertile couples. Urology 2018; 113: 52-8.
        [http://dx.doi.org/10.1016/j.urology.2017.11.050] [PMID: 29287977]

[25]   Cowan FM, Johnson AM, Ashley R, Corey L, Mindel A. Relationship between antibodies to herpes simplex virus (HSV) and symptoms of HSV infection. J Infect Dis 1996; 174(3): 470-5.
        [http://dx.doi.org/10.1093/infdis/174.3.470] [PMID: 8769602]

[26]   Neofytou E, Sourvinos G, Asmarianaki M, Spandidos DA, Makrigiannakis A. Prevalence of human herpes virus types 1–7 in the semen of men attending an infertility clinic and correlation with semen parameters. Fertil Steril 2009; 91(6): 2487-94.
        [http://dx.doi.org/10.1016/j.fertnstert.2008.03.074] [PMID: 18565516]

[27]   Naumenko VA, Kushch AA. [Herpes viruses and male infertility--is there any relationship?]. Vopr Virusol 2013; 58(3): 4-9.
        [PMID: 24006625]

[28]   Gimenes F, Souza RP, Bento JC, *et al.* Male infertility: a public health issue caused by sexually transmitted pathogens. Nat Rev Urol 2014; 11(12): 672-87.
        [http://dx.doi.org/10.1038/nrurol.2014.285] [PMID: 25330794]

[29]   Omarova S, Cannon A, Weiss W, Bruccoleri A, Puccio J. Genital Herpes Simplex Virus—An Updated Review. Adv Pediatr 2022; 69(1): 149-62.
        [http://dx.doi.org/10.1016/j.yapd.2022.03.010] [PMID: 35985707]

[30]   Royer HR, Falk EC, Heidrich SM. Genital herpes beliefs: implications for sexual health. J Pediatr Adolesc Gynecol 2013; 26(2): 109-16.
        [http://dx.doi.org/10.1016/j.jpag.2012.11.007] [PMID: 23337309]

[31]   Schwetz TA, Fauci AS. The extended impact of human immunodeficiency virus/AIDS research. J Infect Dis 2019; 219(1): 6-9.
[PMID: 30165415]

[32]   Casper C, Crane H, Menon M, Money D. HIV/AIDS comorbidities: impact on cancer, noncommunicable diseases, and reproductive health. Washington, DC: Review from The International Bank for Reconstruction and Development / The World Bank 2018.

[33]   Gable L, Gostin LO, Hodge JG Jr. HIV/AIDS, reproductive and sexual health, and the law. Am J Public Health 2008; 98(10): 1779-86.
[http://dx.doi.org/10.2105/AJPH.2008.138669] [PMID: 18703431]

[34]   Ochsendorf FR. Sexually transmitted infections: impact on male fertility. Andrologia 2008; 40(2): 72-5.
[http://dx.doi.org/10.1111/j.1439-0272.2007.00825.x] [PMID: 18336453]

[35]   Liu W, Han R, Wu H, Han D. Viral threat to male fertility. Andrologia 2018; 50(11): e13140.
[http://dx.doi.org/10.1111/and.13140] [PMID: 30569651]

[36]   Luo L, Deng T, Zhao S, *et al.* Association between HIV infection and prevalence of erectile dysfunction: a systematic review and meta-analysis. J Sex Med 2017; 14(9): 1125-32.
[http://dx.doi.org/10.1016/j.jsxm.2017.07.001] [PMID: 28778576]

[37]   Romero-Velez G, Lisker-Cervantes A, Villeda-Sandoval CI, *et al.* Erectile dysfunction among HIV patients undergoing highly active antiretroviral therapy: dyslipidemia as a main risk factor. Sex Med 2014; 2(1): 24-30.
[http://dx.doi.org/10.1002/sm2.25] [PMID: 25356298]

[38]   Dejucq N, Jégou B. Viruses in the mammalian male genital tract and their effects on the reproductive system. Microbiol Mol Biol Rev 2001; 65(2): 208-31.
[http://dx.doi.org/10.1128/MMBR.65.2.208-231.2001] [PMID: 11381100]

[39]   Buchacz K, Rogol AD, Lindsey JC, *et al.* Delayed onset of pubertal development in children and adolescents with perinatally acquired HIV infection. J Acquir Immune Defic Syndr 2003; 33(1): 56-65.
[http://dx.doi.org/10.1097/00126334-200305010-00009] [PMID: 12792356]

[40]   Williams PL, Abzug MJ, Jacobson DL, Jiajia W. Pubertal onset in HIV-infected children in the era of combination antiretroviral treatment. AIDS 2013; 27: 1959.
[http://dx.doi.org/10.1097/QAD.0b013e328361195b] [PMID: 24145244]

[41]   Garolla A, Vitagliano A, Muscianisi F, *et al.* Role of viral infections in testicular cancer etiology: evidence from a systematic review and meta-analysis. Front Endocrinol (Lausanne) 2019; 10: 355.
[http://dx.doi.org/10.3389/fendo.2019.00355] [PMID: 31263452]

[42]   Powles T, Bower M, Nelson M, Oliver R. HIV related testicular cancer.

[43]   Sun D, Cao M, Li H, *et al.* Risk of prostate cancer in men with HIV/AIDS: a systematic review and meta-analysis. Prostate Cancer Prostatic Dis 2021; 24(1): 24-34.
[http://dx.doi.org/10.1038/s41391-020-00268-2] [PMID: 32801354]

[44]   Galvin SR, Cohen MS. The role of sexually transmitted diseases in HIV transmission. Nat Rev Microbiol 2004; 2(1): 33-42.
[http://dx.doi.org/10.1038/nrmicro794] [PMID: 15035007]

[45]   Bhatti AB, Usman M, Kandi V. Current scenario of HIV/AIDS, treatment options, and major challenges with compliance to antiretroviral therapy. Cureus 2016; 8(3): e515.
[http://dx.doi.org/10.7759/cureus.515] [PMID: 27054050]

[46]   Clinic M. https://www.mayoclinic.org/diseases-conditions/menopause/in-depth/hormone-therapy/-rt-20046372

[47]   Hatzimouratidis K, Amar E, Eardley I, *et al.* Guidelines on male sexual dysfunction: erectile

dysfunction and premature ejaculation. Eur Urol 2010; 57(5): 804-14.
[http://dx.doi.org/10.1016/j.eururo.2010.02.020] [PMID: 20189712]

[48]   Aliakbari F, Taghizabet N, Rezaei-Tazangi F, Kharazi Nejad E. Effect of semen washing methods on diminishing the transmission of viral infections in artificial reproductive technology. Journal of Preventive Epidemiology 2021; 6(2): e33.
[http://dx.doi.org/10.34172/jpe.2021.33]

[49]   Sengupta P, Leisegang K, Agarwal A. The impact of COVID-19 on the male reproductive tract and fertility: A systematic review. Arab J Urol 2021; 19(3): 423-36.
[http://dx.doi.org/10.1080/2090598X.2021.1955554] [PMID: 34552795]

[50]   Ajayi A, Akhigbe R, Ram S. Management of COVID-19 among health care givers: an Afro-Asian perspective. Asian J Epidemiol 2021; 14: 11-21.
[http://dx.doi.org/10.3923/aje.2021.11.21]

[51]   Zhou P, Yang XL, Wang XG, *et al.* A pneumonia outbreak associated with a new coronavirus of probable bat origin. Nature 2020; 579(7798): 270-3.
[http://dx.doi.org/10.1038/s41586-020-2012-7] [PMID: 32015507]

[52]   Aitken RJ. COVID-19 and human spermatozoa—Potential risks for infertility and sexual transmission? Andrology 2021; 9(1): 48-52.
[http://dx.doi.org/10.1111/andr.12859] [PMID: 32649023]

[53]   Xu J, Qi L, Chi X, *et al.* Orchitis: a complication of severe acute respiratory syndrome (SARS). Biol Reprod 2006; 74(2): 410-6.
[http://dx.doi.org/10.1095/biolreprod.105.044776] [PMID: 16237152]

[54]   Dutta S, Sengupta P. SARS-CoV-2 and male infertility: possible multifaceted pathology. Reprod Sci 2021; 28(1): 23-6.
[http://dx.doi.org/10.1007/s43032-020-00261-z] [PMID: 32651900]

[55]   Li D, Jin M, Bao P, Zhao W, Zhang S. Clinical characteristics and results of semen tests among men with coronavirus disease 2019. JAMA Network open. 2020; 3: e208292

[56]   Bhattacharya K, Mukhopadhyay LD, Goswami R, *et al.* SARS-CoV-2 infection and human semen: possible modes of contamination and transmission. Middle East Fertil Soc J 2021; 26(1): 18.
[http://dx.doi.org/10.1186/s43043-021-00063-6] [PMID: 34177252]

[57]   Ma L, Xie W, Li D, Shi L, Mao Y, Xiong Y, *et al.* Effect of SARS-CoV-2 infection upon male gonadal function: a single center-based study. MedRxiv 2020; 2020.03.
[http://dx.doi.org/10.1101/2020.03.21.20037267]

[58]   Sengupta P, Dutta S. COVID-19 and hypogonadism: secondary immune responses rule-over endocrine mechanisms. Hum Fertil (Camb) 2021; 1-6.
[PMID: 33439057]

[59]   Blendon RJ, Benson JM, DesRoches CM, Raleigh E, Taylor-Clark K. The public's response to severe acute respiratory syndrome in Toronto and the United States. Clin Infect Dis 2004; 38(7): 925-31.
[http://dx.doi.org/10.1086/382355] [PMID: 15034821]

[60]   Dutta S, Sengupta P. SARS-CoV-2 infection, oxidative stress and male reproductive hormones: can testicular-adrenal crosstalk be ruled-out? J Basic Clin Physiol Pharmacol 2020; 31(6): 20200205.
[http://dx.doi.org/10.1515/jbcpp-2020-0205] [PMID: 32889794]

[61]   Sengupta P, Dutta S. Does SARS-CoV-2 infection cause sperm DNA fragmentation? Possible link with oxidative stress. Eur J Contracept Reprod Health Care 2020; 25(5): 405-6.
[http://dx.doi.org/10.1080/13625187.2020.1787376] [PMID: 32643968]

[62]   Le Tortorec A, Matusali G, Mahé D, *et al.* From ancient to emerging infections: the odyssey of viruses in the male genital tract. Physiol Rev 2020; 100(3): 1349-414.
[http://dx.doi.org/10.1152/physrev.00021.2019] [PMID: 32031468]

[63]   Dutta S, Sandhu N, Sengupta P, Alves MG, Henkel R, Agarwal A. Somatic-immune cells crosstalk in-the-making of testicular immune privilege. Reprod Sci 2022; 29(10): 2707-18.
[http://dx.doi.org/10.1007/s43032-021-00721-0] [PMID: 34580844]

[64]   Sarkar D, Dutta S, Roychoudhury S, Poduval P, Jha NK, Dhal PK, *et al.* Pathogenesis of Viral Infections and Male Reproductive Health: An Evidence-Based Study Oxidative Stress and Toxicity in Reproductive Biology and Medicine: A Comprehensive Update on Male Infertility-Volume One. Springer 2022; pp. 325-43.

[65]   Dutta S, Sengupta P, Chakravarthi S. Testicular immune tolerance and viral infections Translational Autoimmunity. Elsevier 2023; pp. 169-81.
[http://dx.doi.org/10.1016/B978-0-323-85389-7.00022-3]

[66]   Dutta S, Sengupta P, Chakravarthi S. Oxidant-Sensitive Inflammatory Pathways and Male Reproductive Functions Oxidative Stress and Toxicity in Reproductive Biology and Medicine: A Comprehensive Update on Male Infertility-Volume One. Springer 2022; pp. 165-80.
[http://dx.doi.org/10.1007/978-3-030-89340-8_8]

[67]   Jacobo P, Guazzone VA, Theas MS, Lustig L. Testicular autoimmunity. Autoimmun Rev 2011; 10(4): 201-4.
[http://dx.doi.org/10.1016/j.autrev.2010.09.026] [PMID: 20932942]

[68]   Zribi N, Chakroun N, Elleuch H, *et al.* Sperm DNA fragmentation and oxidation are independent of malondialdheyde. Reprod Biol Endocrinol 2011; 9(1): 47.
[http://dx.doi.org/10.1186/1477-7827-9-47] [PMID: 21492479]

[69]   Pecou S, Moinard N, Walschaerts M, Pasquier C, Daudin M, Bujan L. Ribavirin and pegylated interferon treatment for hepatitis C was associated not only with semen alterations but also with sperm deoxyribonucleic acid fragmentation in humans. Fertil Steril. 2009; 91: 933. e17-e22.
[http://dx.doi.org/10.1016/j.fertnstert.2008.07.1755]

[70]   Erpenbach KHJ. Systemic treatment with interferon-α 2B: an effective method to prevent sterility after bilateral mumps orchitis. J Urol 1991; 146(1): 54-6.
[http://dx.doi.org/10.1016/S0022-5347(17)37713-3] [PMID: 2056606]

[71]   Drobnis EZ, Nangia AK, Drobnis EZ, Nangia AK. Antivirals and male reproduction Impacts of Medications on Male Fertility. Cham: Springer 2017; pp. 163-78.
[http://dx.doi.org/10.1007/978-3-319-69535-8_11]

[72]   Lee S, Ives AM, Bertke AS. Herpes simplex virus 1 reactivates from autonomic ciliary ganglia independently from sensory trigeminal ganglia to cause recurrent ocular disease. J Virol 2015; 89(16): 8383-91.
[http://dx.doi.org/10.1128/JVI.00468-15] [PMID: 26041294]

[73]   Meinhardt A, Hedger MP. Immunological, paracrine and endocrine aspects of testicular immune privilege. Mol Cell Endocrinol 2011; 335(1): 60-8.
[http://dx.doi.org/10.1016/j.mce.2010.03.022] [PMID: 20363290]

[74]   Fijak M, Bhushan S, Meinhardt A. The immune privilege of the testis Immune Infertility. Springer 2017; pp. 97-107.
[http://dx.doi.org/10.1007/978-3-319-40788-3_5]

[75]   Archana SS, Selvaraju S, Binsila BK, Arangasamy A, Krawetz SA. Immune regulatory molecules as modifiers of semen and fertility: A review. Mol Reprod Dev 2019; 86(11): 1485-504.
[http://dx.doi.org/10.1002/mrd.23263] [PMID: 31518041]

[76]   Jenabian MA, Costiniuk CT, Mehraj V, *et al.* Immune tolerance properties of the testicular tissue as a viral sanctuary site in ART-treated HIV-infected adults. AIDS 2016; 30(18): 2777-86.
[http://dx.doi.org/10.1097/QAD.0000000000001282] [PMID: 27677162]

[77]   Lorenzo-Redondo R, Fryer HR, Bedford T, *et al.* Persistent HIV-1 replication maintains the tissue reservoir during therapy. Nature 2016; 530(7588): 51-6.

[http://dx.doi.org/10.1038/nature16933] [PMID: 26814962]

[78]   Setchell BP. The testis and tissue transplantation: historical aspects. J Reprod Immunol 1990; 18(1): 1-8.
        [http://dx.doi.org/10.1016/0165-0378(90)90020-7] [PMID: 2213727]

[79]   Sand K. Experiments on the internal secretion of the sexual glands, especially on experimental hermaphroditism. J Physiol 1919; 53(3-4): 257-63.
        [http://dx.doi.org/10.1113/jphysiol.1919.sp001875] [PMID: 16993451]

[80]   Mital P, Kaur G, Dufour JM. Immunoprotective Sertoli cells: making allogeneic and xenogeneic transplantation feasible. Reproduction 2010; 139(3): 495-504.
        [http://dx.doi.org/10.1530/REP-09-0384] [PMID: 19995832]

[81]   Lanza RP, Chick WL. Pancreatic Islet Transplantation: Immunoisolation of pancreatic islets: RG Landes; 1994.

[82]   Fijak M, Bhushan S, Meinhardt A. Immunoprivileged sites: the testis. Methods Mol Biol 2010; 677: 459-70.
        [http://dx.doi.org/10.1007/978-1-60761-869-0_29] [PMID: 20941627]

[83]   Tung KSK, Teuscher C, Meng AL. Autoimmunity to spermatozoa and the testis. Immunol Rev 1981; 55(1): 217-55.
        [http://dx.doi.org/10.1111/j.1600-065X.1981.tb00344.x] [PMID: 7016729]

[84]   Eisele E, Siliciano RF. Redefining the viral reservoirs that prevent HIV-1 eradication. Immunity 2012; 37(3): 377-88.
        [http://dx.doi.org/10.1016/j.immuni.2012.08.010] [PMID: 22999944]

[85]   Schindell BG, Webb AL, Kindrachuk J. Persistence and sexual transmission of filoviruses. Viruses 2018; 10(12): 683.
        [http://dx.doi.org/10.3390/v10120683] [PMID: 30513823]

[86]   Mlera L, Bloom ME. Differential zika virus infection of testicular cell lines. Viruses 2019; 11(1): 42.
        [http://dx.doi.org/10.3390/v11010042] [PMID: 30634400]

[87]   Molina DA, Fernández-Cadena J, Fernández-Cadena T, Cárdenas P, Morey-León G, Armas-Gonzales R, *et al.* A suspected case of SARS-CoV-2 persistence with reactivation. 2020.
        [http://dx.doi.org/10.21203/rs.3.rs-92286/v1]

[88]   Hedger MP. Immunophysiology and pathology of inflammation in the testis and epididymis. J Androl 2011; 32(6): 625-40.
        [http://dx.doi.org/10.2164/jandrol.111.012989] [PMID: 21764900]

[89]   Huang J-M, Huang T-H, Qiu H-Y, Fang X-W, Zhuang T-G, Qiu J-W. Studies on the integration of hepatitis B virus DNA sequence in human sperm chromosomes. Asian J Androl 2002; 4(3): 209-12.
        [PMID: 12364978]

[90]   Wang D, Li LB, Hou ZW, *et al.* The integrated HIV-1 provirus in patient sperm chromosome and its transfer into the early embryo by fertilization. PLoS One 2011; 6(12): e28586.
        [http://dx.doi.org/10.1371/journal.pone.0028586] [PMID: 22194862]

[91]   Davis NF, McGuire BB, Mahon JA, Smyth AE, O'Malley KJ, Fitzpatrick JM. The increasing incidence of mumps orchitis: a comprehensive review. BJU Int 2010; 105(8): 1060-5.
        [http://dx.doi.org/10.1111/j.1464-410X.2009.09148.x] [PMID: 20070300]

[92]   Mital P, Hinton BT, Dufour JM. The blood-testis and blood-epididymis barriers are more than just their tight junctions. Biol Reprod 2011; 84(5): 851-8.
        [http://dx.doi.org/10.1095/biolreprod.110.087452] [PMID: 21209417]

[93]   Yule TD, Montoya GD, Russell LD, Williams TM, Tung KS. Autoantigenic germ cells exist outside the blood testis barrier. J Immunol 1988; 141(4): 1161-7.
        [http://dx.doi.org/10.4049/jimmunol.141.4.1161] [PMID: 3397538]

[94]   Silva RC, Costa GMJ, Lacerda SMSN, *et al.* Germ cell transplantation in felids: a potential approach to preserving endangered species. J Androl 2012; 33(2): 264-76.
[http://dx.doi.org/10.2164/jandrol.110.012898] [PMID: 21597091]

[95]   Tang EI, Robinson CL, Chong CN, Chen S, Cheng CY. A look into the testis as a reservoir for HIV and ZIKV—A reproductive biologist's perspective Spermatogenesis. CRC Press 2018; pp. 183-90.

[96]   Avelino-Silva VI, Alvarenga C, Abreu C, Tozetto-Mendoza TR, Canto CLMd, Manuli ER, *et al.* Potential effect of Zika virus infection on human male fertility? Revist Inst Med Trop São Paulo. 2018; 60.

[97]   Hu B, Liu K, Ruan Y, *et al.* Evaluation of mid- and long-term impact of COVID-19 on male fertility through evaluating semen parameters. Transl Androl Urol 2022; 11(2): 159-67.
[http://dx.doi.org/10.21037/tau-21-922] [PMID: 35280660]

[98]   Smith EM, Ritchie JM, Yankowitz J, Swarnavel S, Wang D, Haugen TH, *et al.* Human papillomavirus prevalence and types in newborns and parents: concordance and modes of transmission. Sex Transmit Dis 2004; pp. 57-62.

[99]   Dekker G, Robillard PY, Roberts C. The etiology of preeclampsia: the role of the father. J Reprod Immunol 2011; 89(2): 126-32.
[http://dx.doi.org/10.1016/j.jri.2010.12.010] [PMID: 21529966]

[100]   Indolfi G, Resti M. Perinatal transmission of hepatitis C virus infection. J Med Virol 2009; 81(5): 836-43.
[http://dx.doi.org/10.1002/jmv.21437] [PMID: 19319981]

[101]   Perino A, Giovannelli L, Schillaci R, *et al.* Human papillomavirus infection in couples undergoing in vitro fertilization procedures: impact on reproductive outcomes. Fertil Steril 2011; 95(5): 1845-8.
[http://dx.doi.org/10.1016/j.fertnstert.2010.11.047] [PMID: 21167483]

[102]   Garolla A, Pizzol D, Bertoldo A, Menegazzo M, Barzon L, Foresta C. Sperm viral infection and male infertility: focus on HBV, HCV, HIV, HPV, HSV, HCMV, and AAV. J Reprod Immunol 2013; 100(1): 20-9.
[http://dx.doi.org/10.1016/j.jri.2013.03.004] [PMID: 23668923]

[103]   Schuppe HC, Pilatz A, Hossain H, Diemer T, Wagenlehner F, Weidner W. Urogenital infection as a risk factor for male infertility. Dtsch Arztebl Int 2017; 114(19): 339-46.
[http://dx.doi.org/10.3238/arztebl.2017.0339] [PMID: 28597829]

[104]   Evans AS. Viral infections of humans: epidemiology and control. Springer Science & Business Media 2013.

[105]   Pellati D, Mylonakis I, Bertoloni G, *et al.* Genital tract infections and infertility. Eur J Obstet Gynecol Reprod Biol 2008; 140(1): 3-11.
[http://dx.doi.org/10.1016/j.ejogrb.2008.03.009] [PMID: 18456385]

[106]   Rivero MJ, Kulkarni N, Thirumavalavan N, Ramasamy R. Evaluation and management of male genital tract infections in the setting of male infertility: an updated review. Curr Opin Urol 2023; 33(3): 180-6.
[http://dx.doi.org/10.1097/MOU.0000000000001081] [PMID: 36861760]

[107]   Gianella S, Strain MC, Rought SE, *et al.* Associations between virologic and immunologic dynamics in blood and in the male genital tract. J Virol 2012; 86(3): 1307-15.
[http://dx.doi.org/10.1128/JVI.06077-11] [PMID: 22114342]

[108]   Narvekar S. Microbiology of Semen and Male Genital Tract Infections. 2013.

[109]   Teixeira TA, Oliveira YC, Bernardes FS, *et al.* Viral infections and implications for male reproductive health. Asian J Androl 2021; 23(4): 335-47.
[http://dx.doi.org/10.4103/aja.aja_82_20] [PMID: 33473014]

[110]   Stanley M. Genital human papillomavirus infections—current and prospective therapies. JNCI

Monogr 2003; pp. 117-24.

[111]   Gupta R, Wald A, Krantz E, *et al.* Valacyclovir and acyclovir for suppression of shedding of herpes simplex virus in the genital tract. J Infect Dis 2004; 190(8): 1374-81.
[http://dx.doi.org/10.1086/424519] [PMID: 15378428]

[112]   Buhles WC Jr, Mastre RJ, Tinker AJ, Strand V, Koretz SH, Koretz SH. Ganciclovir treatment of life- or sight-threatening cytomegalovirus infection: experience in 314 immunocompromised patients. Clin Infect Dis 1988; 10 (Suppl. 3): S495-506.
[http://dx.doi.org/10.1093/clinids/10.Supplement_3.S495] [PMID: 2847286]

[113]   Bergot AS, Kassianos A, Frazer IH, Mittal D. New Approaches to Immunotherapy for HPV Associated Cancers. Cancers (Basel) 2011; 3(3): 3461-95.
[http://dx.doi.org/10.3390/cancers3033461] [PMID: 24212964]

[114]   Caine EA, Scheaffer SM, Arora N, *et al.* Interferon lambda protects the female reproductive tract against Zika virus infection. Nat Commun 2019; 10(1): 280.
[http://dx.doi.org/10.1038/s41467-018-07993-2] [PMID: 30655513]

[115]   Czelusta AJ, Evans T, Arany I, Tyring SK. A guide to immunotherapy of genital warts: focus on interferon and imiquimod. BioDrugs 1999; 11(5): 319-32.
[http://dx.doi.org/10.2165/00063030-199911050-00004] [PMID: 18031142]

[116]   Skeate JG, Woodham AW, Einstein MH, Da Silva DM, Kast WM. Current therapeutic vaccination and immunotherapy strategies for HPV-related diseases. Hum Vaccin Immunother 2016; 12(6): 1418-29.
[http://dx.doi.org/10.1080/21645515.2015.1136039] [PMID: 26835746]

[117]   Schuppe HC, Meinhardt A, Allam JP, Bergmann M, Weidner W, Haidl G. Chronic orchitis: a neglected cause of male infertility? Andrologia 2008; 40(2): 84-91.
[http://dx.doi.org/10.1111/j.1439-0272.2008.00837.x] [PMID: 18336456]

[118]   Yanofsky VR, Patel RV, Goldenberg G. Genital warts: a comprehensive review. J Clin Aesthet Dermatol 2012; 5(6): 25-36.
[PMID: 22768354]

[119]   Le Tortorec A, Matusali G, Mahé D, *et al.* From ancient to emerging infections: the odyssey of viruses in the male genital tract. Physiol Rev 2020; 100(3): 1349-414
[http://dx.doi.org/10.1152/physrev.00021.2019] [PMID: 32031468]

[120]   Grandahl M, Nevéus T. Barriers towards HPV Vaccinations for Boys and Young Men: A Narrative Review. Viruses 2021; 13(8): 1644.
[http://dx.doi.org/10.3390/v13081644] [PMID: 34452508]

[121]   Workowski KA, Bachmann LH, Chan PA, Johnston CM, Muzny CA, Park I, *et al.* Sexually Transmitted Infections Treatment Guidelines, 2021. MMWR Recommendations and reports : Morbidity and mortality weekly report Recommendations and reports. 2021; 70: 1-187.

[122]   Al-Nasiry S, Ambrosino E, Schlaepfer M, *et al.* The Interplay Between Reproductive Tract Microbiota and Immunological System in Human Reproduction. Front Immunol 2020; 11: 378.
[http://dx.doi.org/10.3389/fimmu.2020.00378] [PMID: 32231664]

[123]   Assidi M. Infertility in Men: Advances towards a Comprehensive and Integrative Strategy for Precision Theranostics. Cells 2022; 11(10): 1711.
[http://dx.doi.org/10.3390/cells11101711] [PMID: 35626747]

[124]   Dutta S, Sengupta P, Chakravarthi S. Testicular immune tolerance and viral infections. InTranslational Autoimmunity 2023 Jan 1 (pp. 169-181). Academic Press
[http://dx.doi.org/10.1016/B978-0-323-85389-7.00022-3]

CHAPTER 9

Fungal Infections of the Male Reproductive System

Abstract: The impact of fungal or mycotic infections on male reproductive health, while significant, remains largely underinvestigated compared to other types of infections in the male reproductive tract. Mycotic infections, though less prevalent than their bacterial and viral analogs, carry considerable hazards encompassing fertility impairment, urinary dysfunctions, and general health deterioration. This chapter chiefly concentrates on three distinct fungal species: *Candida albicans, Aspergillus fumigatus*, and *Cryptococcus neoformans*, each of which presents unique pathogenic modalities and clinical complexities. *C. albicans*, customarily a symbiotic organism, can initiate diseases such as balanitis under specific circumstances. Its capacity to form biofilms serves to augment its resistance to antifungal therapy. *A. fumigatus*, an environmental fungus, is predominantly associated with infections that occur as a result of systemic involvement, emphasizing its opportunistic proclivity in states of compromised immunity. *C. neoformans*, primarily associated with immunocompromised conditions like HIV/AIDS, can trigger serious systemic complications, including prostatitis and orchitis. The present chapter stresses the diverse risk factors predisposing individuals to these infections, which include immunosuppression, antibiotic usage that perturbs the regular microbial flora, and certain lifestyle behaviors. Consequently, an exhaustive comprehension of these mycotic pathogens, their pathogenic mechanisms, and their associated risk factors is indispensable for the development of effective prevention, diagnostic, and management strategies. Despite their comparative infrequency, the substantial health implications of these infections mandate rigorous examination and scrutiny.

Keywords: Antifungal Agents, Aspergillus fumigatus, Candida albicans, Cryptococcus neoformans, Differential Diagnosis, Epididymitis, Fungal Diagnostics, Fungal Prostatitis, Genital Candidiasis, Immunocompromised Host, Male Genital Diseases, Mycological Typing Techniques, Mycoses, Orchitis, Penile Diseases, Male Reproductive System, Seminal Vesiculitis, Testicular Diseases, Treatment Outcome, Urogenital Abnormalities, Vas Deferens.

INTRODUCTION

Fungal infections within the male reproductive system, while less widespread compared to bacterial infections, represent a significant component of genitourinary infections [1, 2]. These infections ensue when fungi, which are eukaryotic microbes, establish colonization and undergo proliferation within the

Sulagna Dutta & Pallav Sengupta

anatomical structures of the male reproductive system. This includes the testicles, epididymis, vas deferens, seminal vesicles, prostate gland, and the external genital organs, with a particular emphasis on the penis [3]. Pathogenesis is characterized by the perturbation of the resident microbiota or the weakening of the host's immune defenses, facilitating an environment that is amenable to fungal proliferation [3]. Among the causative agents, species belonging to the Candida genus, most notably *Candida albicans*, are predominantly implicated [4]. Nonetheless, other fungal taxa might also be involved depending on various determinants, such as geographic prevalence and the immunological status of the host. Predisposing factors encompass diabetes mellitus, immunocompromised state, extended administration of antibiotics, and suboptimal personal hygiene [1, 5].

The clinical presentations associated with mycotic infections of the male reproductive system are heterogeneous [6]. The symptomatology may span from inconspicuous irritations to acute inflammations and may encompass pruritus, erythema, a sensation of burning, exudate, and pain [7]. In extreme instances, these infections can exert deleterious consequences on male reproductive competence [8]. The diagnostic procedures for mycotic infections necessitate a comprehensive approach. The clinical evaluation commences with an in-depth patient history and physical examination. Laboratory analyses comprise microscopy, fungal culturing, and, in certain scenarios, molecular techniques such as polymerase chain reaction (PCR) for pinpointing the specific microbial agent. It is crucial to differentiate mycotic infections from other genitourinary infections, as the therapeutic strategies and prognostic outcomes diverge considerably [8].

This chapter explores the complexities of mycotic infections within the male reproductive system, covering aspects of microbial pathogenesis, predisposing factors, clinical manifestations, and diagnostic procedures. Furthermore, it elucidates the potential ramifications of these infections on male reproductive capability and underscores the significance of prompt identification and judicious management.

CAUSES OF FUNGAL INFECTIONS

Fungal infections in the male reproductive system are caused by a variety of fungi. Some of the most common types of fungi that cause these infections include *Candida albicans*, *Aspergillus fumigatus*, and *Cryptococcus neoformans*. These fungi can cause a range of symptoms and can have serious consequences if left untreated [3, 4, 6]. In the following sections, the most common types of fungi that can cause infections in the male reproductive system are discussed, along with the associated risk factors.

Candida Albicans

Candida albicans is a type of yeast that is commonly found in the human body, especially in the gastrointestinal tract and the female reproductive system [4]. However, in certain circumstances, it can also infect the male reproductive system, leading to a range of symptoms and complications [1].

Causes

Candida albicans infections of the male reproductive system can occur for several reasons. One of the most common causes is a weakened immune system. This can happen due to a variety of factors, including chronic diseases like diabetes or human immunodeficiency virus (HIV), the use of immunosuppressive drugs, or lifestyle factors like poor nutrition, lack of sleep, and excessive stress [9]. Another common cause of *Candida albicans* infections of the male reproductive system is the use of antibiotics. Antibiotics kill off not only harmful bacteria but also the beneficial ones that help maintain a healthy balance of microorganisms in the body. This can create an environment in which *Candida albicans* can grow unchecked [10]. Other risk factors for *Candida albicans* infections of the male reproductive system include sexual activity, especially with a partner who has a vaginal yeast infection, and poor hygiene, especially in uncircumcised men. Certain types of clothing, such as tight-fitting pants or underwear made from non-breathable materials, can also create an environment that promotes the growth of *Candida albicans* [3].

Symptoms

The symptoms of *Candida albicans* infections of the male reproductive system can vary depending on the severity of the infection and the area of the reproductive system that is affected. Some of the most common symptoms include redness, itching, and irritation of the glans or foreskin; white, clumpy discharge under the foreskin; painful urination or discomfort during sexual activity; swelling and inflammation of the penis and surrounding tissue; difficulty retracting the foreskin; rash or blisters on the penis or scrotum. In severe cases, *Candida albicans* infections of the male reproductive system can lead to systemic infections, which can cause fever, chills, and other flu-like symptoms [11].

Diagnosis

To diagnose *Candida albicans* infections of the male reproductive system, a doctor will typically perform a physical examination and ask about the patient's symptoms and medical history. They may also take a swab of the affected area to test for the presence of *Candida albicans* or other microorganisms. In some cases, a doctor may also order blood tests or imaging studies to rule out other underlying conditions that may be contributing to the patient's symptoms [5, 11].

Treatment

The treatment of *Candida albicans* infections of the male reproductive system typically involves a combination of antifungal medications and lifestyle changes to reduce the risk of future infections. Antifungal medications may be administered orally or topically, depending on the severity of the infection and the area of the reproductive system that is affected. Some of the most commonly used antifungal medications for *Candida albicans* infections include fluconazole, itraconazole, and clotrimazole. In addition to medications, lifestyle changes can also be helpful in reducing the risk of future *Candida albicans* infections of the male reproductive system. These may include practicing good hygiene, including washing the genital area daily with mild soap and water, avoiding tight-fitting clothing and synthetic fabrics, wearing breathable cotton underwear, and avoiding sexual activity until the infection has cleared [5, 11].

Aspergillus Fumigatus

Aspergillus fumigatus is a ubiquitous mold that is commonly found in soil, water, and decaying organic matter. It is a known human pathogen that can cause various infections, including those of the respiratory, cutaneous, and digestive systems. In rare cases, *Aspergillus fumigatus* infections can also affect the male reproductive system, leading to a range of symptoms and complications [12].

Causes

Aspergillus fumigatus infections of the male reproductive system are relatively rare and occur mainly in individuals with weakened immune systems. These infections can develop through various routes, including hematogenous spread, direct inoculation, or from an adjacent infected site. Hematogenous spread is the most common route of infection, and it occurs when the fungus enters the bloodstream and spreads to other parts of the body, including the male reproductive system. Direct inoculation can occur during medical procedures, such as surgery or biopsy, or as a result of trauma. In rare cases, infections can also develop from an adjacent infected site, such as a urinary tract infection [13].

Symptoms

Aspergillus fumigatus infections of the male reproductive system can present with a wide range of symptoms, depending on the location and extent of the infection. Some of the most common symptoms include:

Pain and swelling in the testicles: These are common symptoms of *Aspergillus fumigatus* infections of the male reproductive system. The pain and swelling can be unilateral or bilateral and may be accompanied by redness and warmth [14].

Discharge from the urethra: This symptom is more commonly associated with infections of the urinary tract. However, in some cases, *Aspergillus fumigatus* infections can also cause discharge from the urethra [14].

Painful urination: Painful urination is a common symptom of infections of the urinary tract. In some cases, *Aspergillus fumigatus* infections can also cause painful urination [14].

Erectile dysfunction: In some cases, *Aspergillus fumigatus* infections can affect the blood supply to the penis, leading to erectile dysfunction [15].

Infertility: *Aspergillus fumigatus* infections can cause damage to the testicles, leading to reduced sperm production and infertility [15].

Diagnosis: The diagnosis of *Aspergillus fumigatus* infections of the male reproductive system can be challenging, as the symptoms can be non-specific and similar to those of other conditions. However, the diagnosis is typically based on a combination of clinical evaluation, imaging studies, and laboratory tests [6, 13, 15]. The following are some of the diagnostic tests that may be used:

Imaging studies: Imaging studies, such as ultrasound, can help identify the presence of abscesses, inflammation, or other abnormalities in the male reproductive system.

Microscopic examination: A sample of the discharge or tissue from the affected area can be examined under a microscope to detect the presence of *Aspergillus fumigatus*.

Fungal culture: A culture can be taken from the affected area to identify the specific type of fungus causing the infection.

Serological tests: Serological tests, such as the detection of specific antibodies or antigens in the blood, can help confirm the diagnosis of *Aspergillus fumigatus* infections.

Treatment Options

The primary treatment for *Aspergillus fumigatus* infections of the male reproductive system is antifungal therapy. The drugs commonly used for this purpose include amphotericin B, itraconazole, voriconazole, and posaconazole.

The choice of antifungal drug depends on various factors such as the severity of the infection, the patient's age, and any underlying medical conditions. It has been implied by various studies that the participation of endogenous protease inhibitors in the mucosal host defense could be considerable. Located on various mucosal surfaces, such as those of the respiratory and genital tracts, Antileukoprotease (ALP), an essential protease inhibitor, is found. The recombinant (r) ALP has been identified to exhibit antimicrobial potential against human fungal pathogens, including *Aspergillus fumigatus* and *Candida albicans* [16]. The duration of antifungal therapy can vary from a few weeks to several months, depending on the extent of the infection and the response to treatment. In some cases, long-term antifungal therapy may be required to prevent a recurrence [17, 18].

In some cases, surgical intervention may be necessary to manage *Aspergillus fumigatus* infections of the male reproductive system [19]. This is particularly true in cases where there is a collection of pus or abscesses that cannot be managed with antibiotics or antifungal therapy alone. Surgical options include drainage of the abscess, debridement of necrotic tissue, or removal of the affected organ. The choice of surgical procedure depends on the extent and severity of the infection, as well as the patient's overall health [20].

In addition to antifungal therapy and surgery, supportive therapy can also be useful in managing *Aspergillus fumigatus* infections of the male reproductive system. This can include pain management, fluid and electrolyte replacement, and nutritional support.

Prognosis

The prognosis for *Aspergillus fumigatus* infections of the male reproductive system depends on various factors, such as the severity of the infection, the response to treatment, and the presence of any underlying medical conditions. In general, early diagnosis and prompt initiation of appropriate therapy can improve the prognosis. However, in some cases, the infection can result in significant morbidity and even mortality, particularly in patients with weakened immune systems [6, 15].

Prevention

Prevention of *Aspergillus fumigatus* infections of the male reproductive system primarily involves avoiding exposure to the fungus. This can be achieved by maintaining good hygiene practices, avoiding environments where the fungus is prevalent, and using appropriate protective equipment when necessary [6, 15].

Cryptococcus Neoformans

Cryptococcus neoformans is a type of fungus that can cause a variety of infections in humans. It is typically found in soil and pigeon droppings and is known for causing lung infections in individuals with weakened immune systems. However, this fungus can also cause infections in other parts of the body, including the male reproductive system. *Cryptococcus neoformans* infections of the male reproductive system are relatively rare, but they can have serious consequences if left untreated [21, 22].

Causes

Cryptococcus neoformans infections of the male reproductive system can occur in individuals with weakened immune systems, such as those with HIV/AIDS or those undergoing chemotherapy [23]. These individuals are at higher risk of developing infections because their immune systems are unable to fight off the fungus effectively. In some cases, *Cryptococcus neoformans* infections of the male reproductive system can occur in healthy individuals. It is believed that these infections are often the result of direct exposure to the fungus, such as through sexual contact with an infected partner [21].

Symptoms

The symptoms of *Cryptococcus neoformans* infections of the male reproductive system can vary depending on the severity of the infection [24, 25]. In some cases, individuals may not experience any symptoms at all. However, when symptoms do occur, they may include pain or discomfort in the testicles or scrotum, swelling or inflammation of the testicles or scrotum, discharge from the penis, and pain or discomfort during urination [24].

Diagnosis

The diagnosis of *Cryptococcus neoformans* infections of the male reproductive system typically involves a physical examination and laboratory tests. During the physical examination, a healthcare provider may examine the genitals and perform a digital rectal exam to check for any signs of inflammation or infection. Laboratory tests may include a urine culture or a semen analysis to detect the presence of the fungus. In some cases, a biopsy of the affected tissue may be necessary to confirm the diagnosis [5, 21, 26].

Treatment

The treatment of *Cryptococcus neoformans* infections of the male reproductive system typically involves antifungal medications. These medications are designed to kill the fungus and prevent it from spreading to other parts of the body. In some cases, surgery may be necessary to remove infected tissue, particularly if the infection has spread to other areas of the body. Additionally, individuals with weakened immune systems may require additional treatment to boost their immune function and reduce their risk of developing further infections [27, 28].

Prevention

Preventing *Cryptococcus neoformans* infections of the male reproductive system typically involves reducing exposure to the fungus. This may include avoiding contact with pigeon droppings and other sources of the fungus, practicing safe sex to reduce the risk of transmission from an infected partner, and maintaining good hygiene to reduce the risk of infection. Individuals with weakened immune systems may also benefit from taking additional precautions to reduce their risk of infection, such as avoiding contact with individuals who are sick and practicing good hand hygiene [5, 23].

DISCUSSION OF THE RISK FACTORS ASSOCIATED WITH FUNGAL INFECTIONS

Mycotic infections present a complex dilemma in human health, with clinical manifestations varying from cutaneous infections, exemplified by tinea pedis, to severe systemic infections, such as invasive aspergillosis, which can be fatal. The epidemiological and pathological aspects of mycotic infections are governed by an array of risk factors that can be segregated into host-associated, environmental, and medical intervention-related categories [29, 30].

Host-associated determinants encompass a plethora of elements related to the intrinsic and adaptive immune responses of an individual [12]. A paramount host-associated determinant is immune suppression. Individuals with a weakened immune system resulting from conditions such as HIV/AIDS, immunosuppressive treatment post-organ transplantation, or hematological malignancies receiving chemotherapy face an escalated risk of invasive mycotic infections [31]. Neutropenia, denoted by a reduction in neutrophil counts, has a significant association with invasive mycotic infections, owing to the critical role neutrophils play in counteracting fungal pathogens. Moreover, individuals with chronic ailments like diabetes mellitus, chronic obstructive pulmonary disease, or those with skin integrity compromise due to injuries or indwelling medical devices are susceptible to fungal colonization and consequent infection [32, 33].

Genetic determinants are also pivotal in influencing vulnerability to mycotic infections. Variations in genes allied with immune responses, such as those encoding pattern recognition receptors like dectin-1, may render individuals more susceptible to fungal pathogens [34]. Furthermore, primary immunodeficiency disorders, for instance, chronic granulomatous disease, result in impaired phagocytic activity and are correlated with a heightened risk of mycotic infections [35, 36].

Environmental determinants considerably influence the likelihood of acquiring mycotic infections. Individuals inhabiting or journeying to regions with a high incidence of endemic fungal infections, such as those caused by *Histoplasma capsulatum* or *Coccidioides immitis*, are at risk [37]. Additionally, exposure to environments contaminated with fungal pathogens, including construction zones or medical facilities, can lead to infections by opportunistic fungi like Aspergillus species. Climate change has been noted to modify the geographical distribution of fungal species, and extreme meteorological events may promote the dissemination and multiplication of fungal pathogens in new habitats [38].

Medical intervention-related factors are also central to comprehending the risks linked to mycotic infections. The development and extensive utilization of broad-spectrum antibiotics have been ironically associated with an upsurge in mycotic infections [39, 40]. The eradication of commensal bacterial flora, which typically curtails fungal colonization through competitive inhibition, facilitates the unchecked growth of fungi. Additionally, invasive medical procedures or devices, such as central venous catheters or mechanical ventilators, can act as entry points for fungi, especially in patients with critical illnesses. Thus, the risk determinants pertinent to mycotic infections are multifactorial and frequently interconnected. The immune competency, genetic predispositions, environmental exposures, and medical interventions of an individual play substantial roles in dictating susceptibility to mycotic infections [41, 42]. To alleviate the impact of these infections, it is imperative to identify and address these risk determinants through prophylactic strategies, specialized pharmaceutical interventions, and public health initiatives [3, 5, 30, 43].

CONCLUSION

Fungal infections, though less common than bacterial and viral infections, present significant risks to the male reproductive system. They can affect fertility, urinary function, and overall health. The predominant fungi causing infections in the male reproductive system include Candida albicans, Aspergillus fumigatus, and Cryptococcus neoformans. Each of these presents unique clinical challenges and has different pathogenic mechanisms:

Candida albicans is a commensal organism that, under certain conditions, can become pathogenic and cause infections such as balanitis. It is noteworthy for its ability to form biofilms, which can contribute to its resistance to antifungal agents. Aspergillus fumigatus, a ubiquitous environmental fungus, can cause systemic infections. Infections in the male reproductive system are typically secondary to a systemic infection, suggesting an opportunistic behavior in immunocompromised patients. Cryptococcus neoformans, often associated with immunocompromised states like HIV/AIDS, can cause severe systemic infections, including meningitis, and may also infect the male reproductive system, leading to complications such as prostatitis and orchitis.

There are several risk factors associated with fungal infections in the male reproductive system. They include immunosuppression (due to conditions like diabetes, HIV/AIDS, or immunosuppressive treatment), antibiotic use (which can disrupt normal microbial flora), and certain lifestyle factors (such as poor hygiene or unprotected sex). Thus, understanding the types of fungi that can cause infections in the male reproductive system, along with their pathogenic mechanisms and the risk factors associated with these infections, is crucial for effective prevention, diagnosis, and treatment. Despite their rarity compared to other types of infections, fungal infections in the male reproductive system can have significant health implications and, therefore, merit careful attention.

REFERENCES

[1]   Pellati D, Mylonakis I, Bertoloni G, *et al.* Genital tract infections and infertility. Eur J Obstet Gynecol Reprod Biol 2008; 140(1): 3-11.
       [http://dx.doi.org/10.1016/j.ejogrb.2008.03.009] [PMID: 18456385]

[2]   Brown GD, Denning DW, Gow NAR, Levitz SM, Netea MG, White TC. Hidden killers: human fungal infections. Sci Transl Med 2012; 4(165): 165rv13.
       [http://dx.doi.org/10.1126/scitranslmed.3004404] [PMID: 23253612]

[3]   Workowski KA, Bachmann LH, Chan PA, Johnston CM, Muzny CA, Park I, *et al.*   Sexually Transmitted Infections Treatment Guidelines, 2021. MMWR Recommendations and reports : Morbidity and mortality weekly report Recommendations and reports. 2021; 70: 1-187.

[4]   Tian YH, Xiong JW, Hu L, Huang DH, Xiong CL. *Candida albicans* and filtrates interfere with human spermatozoal motility and alter the ultrastructure of spermatozoa: an in vitro study. Int J Androl 2007; 30(5): 421-9.
       [http://dx.doi.org/10.1111/j.1365-2605.2006.00734.x] [PMID: 17298548]

[5]   Wise GJ, Talluri GS, Marella VK. Fungal infections of the genitourinary system: manifestations, diagnosis, and treatment. Urol Clin North Am 1999; 26(4): 701-718, vii.
       [http://dx.doi.org/10.1016/S0094-0143(05)70212-3] [PMID: 10584612]

[6]   Sobel JD, Vazquez JA. Fungal infections of the urinary tract. World J Urol 1999; 17(6): 410-4.
       [http://dx.doi.org/10.1007/s003450050167] [PMID: 10654372]

[7]   Aridogan IA, Izol V, Ilkit M. Superficial fungal infections of the male genitalia: A review. Crit Rev Microbiol 2011; 37(3): 237-44.
       [http://dx.doi.org/10.3109/1040841X.2011.572862] [PMID: 21668404]

[8]   Casey HW, Irving GW. Bacterial, Mycoplasmal, Mycotic, and Immune-Mediated Diseases of the Urogenital System. In: Foster HL, Small JD, Fox JG, Eds. Diseases. Academic Press 1982; pp. 43-53.
       [http://dx.doi.org/10.1016/B978-0-12-262502-2.50010-9]

[9]   Castrillón-Duque EX, Puerta Suárez J, Cardona Maya WD. Yeast and Fertility: Effects of *In Vitro*

Activity of *Candida* spp. on Sperm Quality. J Reprod Infertil 2018; 19(1): 49-55.
[PMID: 29850447]

[10]   Liversedge NH, Jenkins JM, Keay SD, *et al.* Antibiotic treatment based on seminal cultures from asymptomatic male partners in *in-vitro* fertilization is unnecessary and may be detrimental. Hum Reprod 1996; 11(6): 1227-31.
[http://dx.doi.org/10.1093/oxfordjournals.humrep.a019361] [PMID: 8671429]

[11]   Pandya I, Shinojia M, Vadukul D, Marfatia YS. Approach to balanitis/balanoposthitis: Current guidelines. Indian J Sex Transm Dis AIDS 2014; 35(2): 155-7.
[http://dx.doi.org/10.4103/0253-7184.142415] [PMID: 26396455]

[12]   Luo Y, Liu F, Deng L, *et al.* Innate and Adaptive Immune Responses Induced by Aspergillus fumigatus Conidia and Hyphae. Curr Microbiol 2023; 80(1): 28.
[http://dx.doi.org/10.1007/s00284-022-03102-1] [PMID: 36474044]

[13]   Singal A, Grover C, Pandhi D, Das S, Jain B. Nosocomial urinary tract aspergilloma in an immunocompetent host: An unusual occurrence. Indian J Dermatol 2013; 58(5): 408.
[http://dx.doi.org/10.4103/0019-5154.117346] [PMID: 24082213]

[14]   Martínez-Salas AJ, Aquino-Matus JE, López-Vejar CE, Gutiérrez Díaz Ceballos ME, Noyola-Guadarrama A. Localized genitourinary tract *Aspergillus* infection in an immunocompetent patient: Bladder and epidymal aspergillosis. Urol Case Rep 2022; 42: 102012.
[http://dx.doi.org/10.1016/j.eucr.2022.102012] [PMID: 35145874]

[15]   Swilaiman SS, O'Gorman CM, Du W, *et al.* Global Sexual Fertility in the Opportunistic Pathogen *Aspergillus fumigatus* and Identification of New Supermater Strains. J Fungi (Basel) 2020; 6(4): 258.
[http://dx.doi.org/10.3390/jof6040258] [PMID: 33143051]

[16]   Tomee JFC, Hiemstra PS, Heinzel-Wieland R, Kauffman HF. Antileukoprotease: an endogenous protein in the innate mucosal defense against fungi. J Infect Dis 1997; 176(3): 740-7.
[http://dx.doi.org/10.1086/514098] [PMID: 9291323]

[17]   Ludwig M, Schneider H, Lohmeyer J, *et al.* Systemic aspergillosis with predominant genitourinary manifestations in an immunocompetent man: what we can learn from a disastrous follow-up. Infection 2005; 33(2): 90-2.
[http://dx.doi.org/10.1007/s15010-005-4070-z] [PMID: 15827878]

[18]   Wise GJ, Shteynshlyuger A. How to diagnose and treat fungal infections in chronic prostatitis. Curr Urol Rep. 2006 Aug;7(4):320-8
[http://dx.doi.org/10.1007/s11934-996-0012-2] [PMID: 16930504]

[19]   González-Vicent M, Lassaletta A, López-Pino MA, Romero-Tejada JC, De La Fuente-Trabado M, Díaz MÁ. *Aspergillus* "fungus ball" of the bladder after hematopoietic transplantation in a pediatric patient: Successful treatment with intravesical voriconazole and surgery. Pediatr Transplant 2008; 12(2): 242-5.
[http://dx.doi.org/10.1111/j.1399-3046.2007.00871.x] [PMID: 18266800]

[20]   Sakamoto S, Ogata J, Salazaki Y, Yoshilado S, Ikegami K. Fungus ball formation of aspergillus in the bladder. an unusual case report. Eur Urol 1978; 4(5): 388-9.
[http://dx.doi.org/10.1159/000474000] [PMID: 710472]

[21]   Guess TE, Rosen JA, McClelland EE. An Overview of Sex Bias in *C. neoformans* Infections. J Fungi (Basel) 2018; 4(2): 49.
[http://dx.doi.org/10.3390/jof4020049] [PMID: 29670032]

[22]   Manfredi R, Rezza G, Coronado VG, *et al.* Is AIDS-related cryptococcosis more frequent among men? AIDS 1995; 9(4): 397-8.
[http://dx.doi.org/10.1097/00002030-199504000-00014] [PMID: 7794547]

[23]   Rapp RP. Changing strategies for the management of invasive fungal infections. Pharmacotherapy 2004; 24(2P2): 4S-28S.

[http://dx.doi.org/10.1592/phco.24.3.4S.33151] [PMID: 14992487]

[24] Martinez LR, Garcia-Rivera J, Casadevall A. Cryptococcus neoformans var. neoformans (serotype D) strains are more susceptible to heat than C. neoformans var. grubii (serotype A) strains. J Clin Microbiol 2001; 39(9): 3365-7.
[http://dx.doi.org/10.1128/JCM.39.9.3365-3367.2001] [PMID: 11526180]

[25] Neafie RC, Marty AM. Unusual infections in humans. Clin Microbiol Rev 1993; 6(1): 34-56.
[http://dx.doi.org/10.1128/CMR.6.1.34] [PMID: 8457979]

[26] Sorrell TC, Chen SCA, Phillips P, Marr KA. Clinical perspectives on Cryptococcus neoformans and Cryptococcus gattii: implications for diagnosis and management. Cryptococcus: from human pathogen to model yeast. Wiley 2010; pp. 595-606.

[27] McClelland EE, Hobbs LM, Rivera J, *et al.* The role of host gender in the pathogenesis of Cryptococcus neoformans infections. PLoS One 2013; 8(5): e63632.
[http://dx.doi.org/10.1371/journal.pone.0063632] [PMID: 23741297]

[28] Egbe CA, Omoregie R, Alex-Ighodalo O. 'Cryptococcus neoformans' infection among human immunodeficiency virus patients on highly active antiretroviral therapy in Benin City, Nigeria. New Zealand J Med Lab Sci 2015; 69: 21-3.

[29] Yoon HJ, Choi HY, Kim YK, Song YJ, Ki M. Prevalence of fungal infections using National Health Insurance data from 2009-2013. South Korea: Epidemiol Heal 2014; p. 36.

[30] Gould D. Diagnosis, prevention and treatment of fungal infections. Nurs Stand 2011; 25(33): 38-48.
[http://dx.doi.org/10.7748/ns.25.33.38.s53] [PMID: 21661530]

[31] Lortholary O, Dupont B. Fungal infections among Patients with AIDS Essentials of Clinical Mycology. Springer 2010; pp. 525-36.

[32] Halsey ES, Rasnake MS, Hospenthal DR. Coccidioidomycosis of the male reproductive tract. Mycopathologia 2005; 159(2): 199-204.
[http://dx.doi.org/10.1007/s11046-004-6260-0] [PMID: 15770443]

[33] Thomas L. and Tracy CR. Treatment of fungal urinary tract infection. Urol Clin 2015; 42(4): 473-43
[http://dx.doi.org/10.1016/j.ucl.2015.05.010] [PMID: 26475944]

[34] Chen SM, Shen H, Zhang T, *et al.* Dectin-1 plays an important role in host defense against systemic *Candida glabrata* infection. Virulence 2017; 8(8): 1643-56.
[http://dx.doi.org/10.1080/21505594.2017.1346756] [PMID: 28658592]

[35] Cohen MS, Isturiz RE, Malech HL, *et al.* Fungal infection in chronic granulomatous disease. Am J Med 1981; 71(1): 59-66.
[http://dx.doi.org/10.1016/0002-9343(81)90259-X] [PMID: 7195647]

[36] Anjani G, Vignesh P, Joshi V, *et al.* Recent advances in chronic granulomatous disease. Genes Dis 2020; 7(1): 84-92.
[http://dx.doi.org/10.1016/j.gendis.2019.07.010] [PMID: 32181279]

[37] Walsh TJ, Groll AH. Emerging fungal pathogens: evolving challenges to immunocompromised patients for the twenty-first century. Transpl Infect Dis 1999; 1(4): 247-61.
[http://dx.doi.org/10.1034/j.1399-3062.1999.010404.x] [PMID: 11428996]

[38] Gnat S, Łagowski D, Nowakiewicz A, Dyląg M. A global view on fungal infections in humans and animals: infections caused by dimorphic fungi and dermatophytoses. J Appl Microbiol 2021; 131(6): 2688-704.
[http://dx.doi.org/10.1111/jam.15084] [PMID: 33754409]

[39] Maertens J, Vrebos M, Boogaerts M. Assessing risk factors for systemic fungal infections. Eur J Cancer Care (Engl) 2001; 10(1): 56-62.
[http://dx.doi.org/10.1046/j.1365-2354.2001.00241.x] [PMID: 11827268]

[40] Salehi M, Ahmadikia K, Badali H, Khodavaisy S. Opportunistic fungal infections in the epidemic area

of COVID-19: a clinical and diagnostic perspective from Iran. Mycopathologia 2020; 185(4): 607-11.
[http://dx.doi.org/10.1007/s11046-020-00472-7] [PMID: 32737746]

[41]   Enoch DA, Ludlam HA, Brown NM. Invasive fungal infections: a review of epidemiology and management options. J Med Microbiol 2006; 55(7): 809-18.
[http://dx.doi.org/10.1099/jmm.0.46548-0] [PMID: 16772406]

[42]   Brunke S, Mogavero S, Kasper L, Hube B. Virulence factors in fungal pathogens of man. Curr Opin Microbiol 2016; 32: 89-95.
[http://dx.doi.org/10.1016/j.mib.2016.05.010] [PMID: 27257746]

[43]   Richardson MD, Warnock DW. Fungal infection: diagnosis and management. John Wiley & Sons 2012.
[http://dx.doi.org/10.1002/9781118321492]

CHAPTER 10

Male Reproductive Tract Infections: Diagnosis and Treatment in Relation to Male Infertility

Abstract: Male reproductive tract infections (MRTIs) are a notable yet frequently overlooked contributor to male infertility. The complex interplay between infections and the male reproductive capacity stems from both direct and indirect effects these infections exert on sperm functionality, quality, and the seminal milieu. This chapter provides an exhaustive examination of the identification and management of MRTIs in relation to male infertility. Cutting-edge diagnostic methods, encompassing semen evaluation, molecular identification, and imaging techniques, have markedly elevated the detection precision for causative agents and facilitated a thorough understanding of how infections impact male reproductive wellness. Essential pathogens highlighted include bacteria, viruses, and occasionally parasites, each leaving distinct pathological footprints on the male reproductive apparatus. The chapter also emphasizes the need for tailored therapeutic approaches, balancing the advantages of antibiotics, antivirals, and supplementary treatments against potential risks to male fertility. Moreover, the indirect repercussions of MRTIs, such as the production of reactive oxygen species and immune reactions, are explored to shed light on the diverse influence of these infections. Given the escalating concerns surrounding antibiotic resistance and the associated threats to male reproductive wellbeing, this section champions a discerning treatment methodology. As comprehension of the interrelation between MRTIs and male infertility expands, this chapter is invaluable for medical practitioners, researchers, and scholars aiming for improved patient results in male reproductive health.

Keywords: Andrology, Antibiotics, Assisted reproductive techniques, Anti-inflammatory agents, Antioxidants, Azooospermia, Chlamydia Infections, Epididymitis, Gonorrhea, Male Infertility, Male Genital Diseases, Mycoplasma Infections, Orchitis, Prostatitis, Semen Analysis, Sperm Motility, Sperm Count, Spermatozoa, Urethritis, Urine analysis, Urogenital Infections.

INTRODUCTION

Within the sphere of human fertility, it becomes vital to understand the implications of infections within the male genital tract, along with their management, due to their significant impact on male reproductive capabilities [1]. Male reproductive tract infections (MRTIs), often trivialized, possess the ability to generate grave consequences by undermining the efficacy of the male reproductive system, modifying the quality of sperm cells, and resulting in infertility associated with male factors [2].

Male infertility accounts for approximately 50% of all cases of infertility and is typified by a plethora of contributing factors [3]. A significant correlation between MRTIs and male infertility has been established, revealing a complex and sophisticated interaction. Pathogens, including bacteria, viruses, and parasites, can have a direct effect on sperm production and sperm cell functionality or induce obstructions in the male genital tract, thus hindering fertilization [2]. Chronic infections can cause sustained damage, resulting in compromised semen quality and, in specific instances, an absence of sperm in the semen (azoospermia). Additionally, the systemic inflammatory response provoked by these pathogens can augment the pathological mechanisms underlying male infertility [4].

The aim of this chapter is to scrupulously analyze the nuances of diagnosing and managing MRTIs in the context of male infertility. Our ambition is to provide a comprehensive understanding of the pathophysiological mechanisms through which infections detrimentally affect male fertility and to scrutinize the therapeutic approaches used to combat these maladies. By delving into the latest advancements in this field, this chapter seeks to enhance understanding of the importance of MRTIs in male infertility, highlighting the urgency for timely diagnosis and effective treatment. We are hopeful that this insight will lay the foundation for improvements in patient care and foster advancements in the field of male reproductive health.

DIAGNOSIS OF MALE REPRODUCTIVE TRACT INFECTIONS

Male reproductive tract infections can affect different parts of the male reproductive system, including the urethra, testes, epididymis, prostate, and seminal vesicles [5]. These infections can cause a range of symptoms, including pain, discomfort, and swelling, and can lead to infertility and other serious complications if left untreated. Diagnosing male reproductive tract infections can be challenging, as many of the symptoms can be non-specific and overlap with other conditions. The diagnosis of male reproductive tract infections often involves a combination of physical examination, medical history, and laboratory tests [6, 7].

Physical Examination

A physical examination is usually the first step in diagnosing male reproductive tract infections. During this examination, the physician will check for any visible signs of infection, such as redness, swelling, or discharge. The physician will also feel for any lumps, bumps, or abnormalities in the genital area [8]. The patient's medical history is also an essential component of the examination. The physician may ask about symptoms, past sexual activity, and any history of sexually transmitted infections (STIs) [9].

During the physical examination, the physician may also perform a digital rectal exam (DRE). This is a physical examination of the prostate gland, which is located just below the bladder and in front of the rectum [10]. The physician will insert a gloved, lubricated finger into the rectum to feel for any abnormalities, such as tenderness, swelling, or lumps. The prostate gland can become inflamed or infected, leading to a condition called prostatitis. Symptoms of prostatitis can include pain in the lower back or groin, difficulty urinating, and pain during ejaculation. In addition to the DRE, the physician may also perform a urethral swab. This involves inserting a small, flexible swab into the urethra to collect a sample of discharge or cells for laboratory analysis. A urethral swab can help diagnose a variety of infections, including chlamydia, gonorrhea, and other bacterial infections [10, 11].

The physician may also perform a testicular exam during the physical examination Fig. (**11**). This involves feeling each testicle to check for any abnormalities, such as lumps or swelling. Testicular cancer is a relatively rare but serious condition that can cause swelling or lumps in the testicles [12]. The physician may also check for varicoceles, which are enlarged veins in the scrotum that can affect sperm production [13]. Another aspect of the physical examination is to check for any skin lesions, which can be a sign of infection or other conditions such as skin cancer. The physician will also look for any signs of swelling, tenderness, or pain in the groin or pelvic area. The physician may also ask the patient to cough or perform a Valsalva maneuver, which involves bearing down as if having a bowel movement, to check for any signs of hernias [12].

Medical History

The diagnosis of male reproductive tract infections begins with a thorough medical history of the patient. The medical history provides the clinician with important information that can help in identifying potential risk factors, determining the duration of symptoms, and pinpointing the likely etiology of the infection [14]. The medical history of the patient should include a detailed description of the presenting symptoms, including the onset, duration, severity, and progression of the infection. Patients with a suspected male reproductive tract infection typically present with symptoms such as pain, discharge, and difficulty urinating. The location and severity of the pain should be noted, along with any associated symptoms such as fever or chills. The clinician should also ask about the sexual history of the patient, including the number of sexual partners, the frequency of sexual activity, and any recent unprotected sexual encounters. Sexual history is a crucial component of medical history since most male reproductive tract infections are sexually transmitted. Patients who engage in high-risk sexual behavior, such as having multiple sexual partners, are at a higher risk of developing a sexually transmitted infection [8].

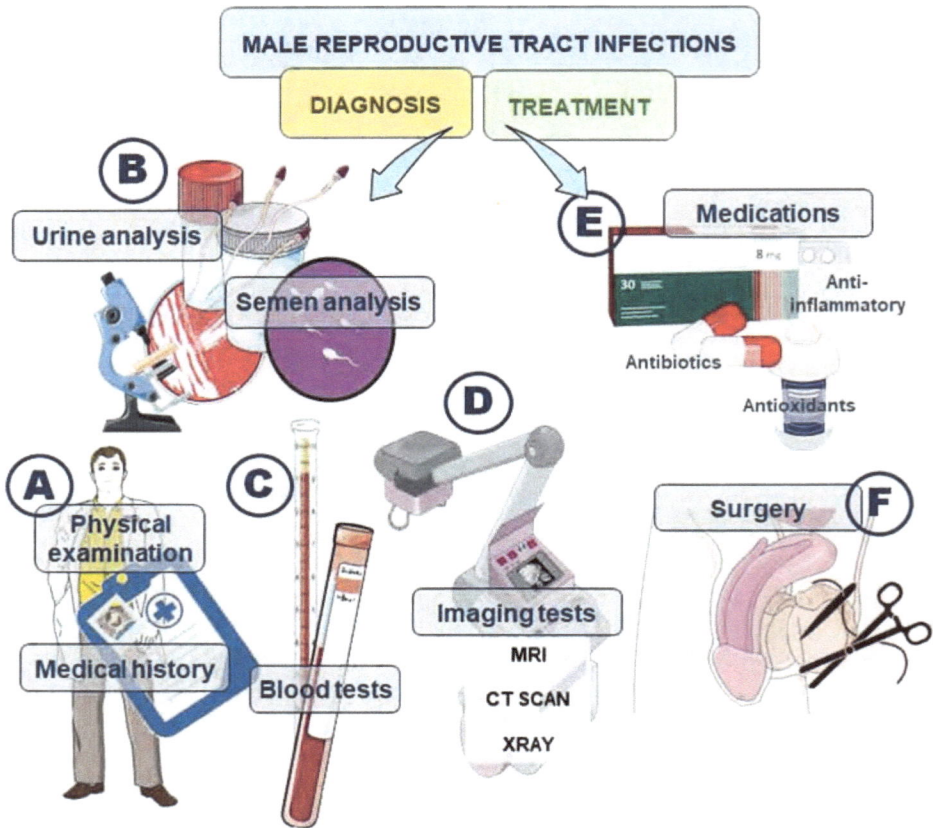

Fig. (11). Common diagnostic and treatment regimen followed for male reproductive tract infections.

In addition to sexual history, the clinician should also ask about the medical history of the patient, including any pre-existing medical conditions or recent surgeries. Patients with underlying medical conditions such as diabetes are at an increased risk of developing infections, including those of the male reproductive tract. The clinician should also inquire about the use of medications or other substances that may contribute to the development of male reproductive tract infections. Certain medications, such as antibiotics, can disrupt the normal flora of the male reproductive tract, making it more susceptible to infections. Additionally, recreational drugs such as cocaine and methamphetamine have been associated with an increased risk of sexually transmitted infections [14].

Other factors that may be relevant to the diagnosis of male reproductive tract infections include the occupation and lifestyle habits of the patient. For example, patients who work in environments with exposure to certain chemicals or toxins may be at an increased risk of developing infections. Similarly, lifestyle habits such as smoking or excessive alcohol consumption may weaken the immune system, making the patient more susceptible to infections [12, 15].

Laboratory Tests

Urine Culture

One common diagnostic tool used in the diagnosis of male reproductive tract infections is a urine culture Fig. (**11**). A urine culture is a laboratory test that is used to identify and isolate bacteria present in a urine sample. This test is performed to detect bacterial infections in the urinary tract, which can include infections of the bladder, urethra, and prostate [16]. In the case of male reproductive tract infections, a urine culture can be used to detect bacterial infections in the prostate gland or seminal vesicles. To perform a urine culture, a sample of urine is collected from the patient and sent to a laboratory. The laboratory technician will then spread the urine sample onto a petri dish containing a nutrient-rich agar medium. The dish is then incubated at a specific temperature for a certain amount of time to allow any bacteria present in the sample to grow and multiply. After the incubation period, the technician will examine the petri dish for the presence of bacterial colonies. If bacterial colonies are present, the technician will then perform further tests to identify the type of bacteria that is causing the infection. This is important because different types of bacteria require different types of antibiotics to treat the infection effectively [16]. A urine culture is a relatively simple and non-invasive test, making it a popular diagnostic tool for male reproductive tract infections. However, there are a few factors to keep in mind when performing and interpreting the results of a urine culture. Firstly, it is important to collect the urine sample properly. The patient should first clean their genital area with a mild soap and warm water before collecting the sample midstream. This means that the patient should start urinating and then collect a sample of urine midstream rather than collecting the first or last part of the urine stream. Secondly, it is important to interpret the results of a urine culture in conjunction with other diagnostic tests and the patient's symptoms.

While a urine culture can identify the presence of bacterial infections, it cannot distinguish between active infections and dormant bacteria that are not causing any symptoms. Therefore, it is important to take into account the patient's clinical presentation and other diagnostic tests, such as a prostate exam or blood tests, when diagnosing male reproductive tract infections. Thirdly, it is important to consider the possibility of false-negative or false-positive results. False-negative results can occur if the bacterial infection is not severe enough to be detected by the urine culture or if the patient has already started taking antibiotics before the test is performed. False-positive results can occur if the urine sample is contaminated during collection or if the patient has a non-bacterial infection. Thus, a urine culture is a useful diagnostic tool in the diagnosis of male reproductive tract infections. It is a relatively simple and non-invasive test that can identify the presence of bacterial infections in the urinary tract, including the prostate gland and seminal vesicles. However, it is important to collect the urine sample properly, interpret the results in conjunction with other diagnostic tests and the patient's symptoms, and consider the possibility of false-negative or false-positive results. With these factors in mind, a urine culture can be an effective tool in diagnosing and treating male reproductive tract infections [16, 17].

Semen Analysis

Semen analysis is a laboratory test that is used to evaluate the health and fertility of a man's semen Fig. (**11**). It is often used as part of a comprehensive evaluation of male reproductive health, especially in cases of infertility or suspected infections. The procedure involves collecting a semen sample and analyzing it for several key parameters, including semen volume, sperm count, sperm motility, and sperm morphology. The results of the analysis can provide important information about the reproductive health of the patient and his chances of fathering a child [5, 8].

Preparing for Semen Analysis

To ensure accurate results, it is important for men to follow certain guidelines when preparing for semen analysis. These guidelines may vary depending on the laboratory where the test is being performed, but some common recommendations include: (a) abstaining from sexual activity for two to five days prior to the test to allow for the build-up of sperm in the semen; (b) avoiding ejaculation through sexual activity or masturbation for at least two days before the test. This helps to ensure that the semen sample contains an adequate number of sperm; (c) not using any lubricants or spermicides during sexual activity or masturbation, as these substances can interfere with semen quality and affect the results of the analysis [18].

Collecting a Semen Sample

Semen samples are usually collected by masturbation, although other methods, such as using a special condom during sexual activity, may also be used. When collecting a semen sample, it is important to follow proper hygiene practices to minimize the risk of contamination. This may include washing the hands and genitals thoroughly with soap and warm water before collecting the sample. Once the semen sample has been collected, it should be brought to the laboratory as soon as possible. The sample should be kept at body temperature during transport and should not be exposed to extreme heat or cold [18, 19].

Interpreting Semen Analysis Results

Semen analysis results are typically reported within a few days of the test. The results may be reported as numerical values or as a narrative description, depending on the laboratory practices. Some of the key parameters that are evaluated during semen analysis include [20]:

Semen Volume

This refers to the amount of semen that is produced during ejaculation. Normal semen volume is typically between 1.5 and 5 milliliters (ml).

Sperm Count

This is a measure of the number of sperm present in the semen sample. A normal sperm count is generally considered to be greater than 15 million sperm per milliliter.

Sperm Motility

This refers to the ability of sperm to move and swim in a forward direction. Normal sperm motility is typically greater than 40%.

Sperm Morphology

This is an assessment of the size and shape of sperm cells. Normal sperm morphology is generally considered to be greater than 4%.

Other parameters that may be evaluated during semen analysis include the pH of the semen, the presence of white blood cells or bacteria, and the level of fructose or other chemicals that are present in the semen.

In general, the results of semen analysis are used to evaluate male fertility and diagnose potential reproductive health problems. Abnormal results may indicate the presence of an infection, hormonal imbalances, or other health issues that may be affecting male fertility. In some cases, further testing or treatment may be recommended based on the results of the analysis.

Blood Tests

Blood tests are commonly used as part of the diagnostic process for male reproductive tract infections [16]. These tests can provide valuable information about the presence of infection, as well as the severity and type of infection that may be present. There are several different types of blood tests that may be used in the diagnosis of male reproductive tract infections, each of which can provide unique insights into the nature of the infection [16]. One of the most common blood tests used in the diagnosis of male reproductive tract infections is the white blood cell count. White blood cells are a critical part of the immune response, and an increase in their numbers in the blood can indicate the presence of infection. Infections in the male reproductive tract can lead to an increase in white blood cell count in the blood as the immune system ramps up its efforts to fight off the infection. A high white blood cell count may indicate the presence of an infection in the prostate, testes, or other parts of the reproductive tract [21]. Another blood test that may be used in the diagnosis of male reproductive tract infections is the erythrocyte sedimentation rate (ESR) test. This test measures the rate at which red blood cells settle in a test tube over a set period of time. When there is an infection or inflammation in the body, the ESR tends to be elevated. In the case of male reproductive tract infections, an elevated ESR may be an indication of an ongoing infection or inflammation in the reproductive tract. In addition to the white blood cell count and ESR tests, there are several other blood tests that may be used in the diagnosis of male reproductive tract infections. For example, the C-reactive protein (CRP) test can be used to measure the level of a specific protein in the blood that is produced in response to inflammation [22]. Like the ESR, an elevated CRP level can indicate the presence of an infection or inflammation in the body. There are also specific blood tests that can be used to identify the presence of certain infections. For example, a blood test for human immunodeficiency virus (HIV) can be used to determine whether a person is infected with this virus, which can lead to a number of different health problems, including infections in the male reproductive tract. Other blood tests that may be used to diagnose infections in the reproductive tract include tests for chlamydia, gonorrhea, and syphilis [22, 23].

It is important to note that while blood tests can be useful in the diagnosis of male reproductive tract infections, they are not always definitive. For example, a man may have an infection in the reproductive tract that does not cause an increase in white blood cells or other inflammatory markers in the blood. In some cases, the presence of an infection may be confirmed only through other diagnostic tests, such as a urine test, semen analysis, or a physical examination. In addition to their use in the diagnosis of male reproductive tract infections, blood tests can also be used to monitor the progression of an infection or the effectiveness of treatment [16]. For example, a man with a confirmed infection in the reproductive tract may have his white blood cell count or ESR monitored over time to determine whether the infection is getting better or worse. Similarly, blood tests may be used to monitor the response to antibiotic therapy or other treatments for infections in the reproductive tract. Thus, blood tests are an important tool in the diagnosis of male reproductive tract infections. These tests can provide valuable information about the presence and nature of an infection, as well as the effectiveness of treatment [24]. However, it is important to note that blood tests are not always definitive, and other diagnostic tests may be needed to confirm the presence of an infection in the reproductive tract.

Imaging Tests

Imaging tests play a crucial role in the diagnosis of male reproductive tract infections. These tests can provide valuable information regarding the condition of the male reproductive system and help in the identification of any potential abnormalities or infections [25].

Ultrasonography

Ultrasonography, also known as ultrasound, is a commonly used imaging test to diagnose male reproductive tract infections [26]. This test uses high-frequency sound waves to create images of the internal organs and tissues. Ultrasonography is a non-invasive test that is performed externally by applying a special gel to the skin and using a transducer to emit sound waves. Ultrasonography can help in the diagnosis of various male reproductive tract infections, including epididymitis, orchitis, prostatitis, and abscesses. This test can also identify any abnormalities in the size, shape, and structure of the male reproductive organs, such as cysts or tumors [25].

Magnetic Resonance Imaging (MRI)

Magnetic resonance imaging (MRI) is another imaging test that can be used to diagnose male reproductive tract infections. This test uses a magnetic field and radio waves to produce detailed images of the internal organs and tissues. MRI is a non-invasive test that can provide more detailed images than ultrasonography. MRI can help in the diagnosis of various male reproductive tract infections, including prostatitis, epididymitis, and testicular cancer. This test can also identify ed by a diversity of pathogens, including ba any abnormalities in the size, shape, and structure of the male reproductive organs, such as cysts or tumors [25].

Computed Tomography (CT)

Computed tomography (CT) is a type of imaging test that uses X-rays to produce detailed images of the internal organs and tissues. This test can provide a more detailed image of the male reproductive tract than ultrasonography, but it also exposes the patient to radiation. CT can help in the diagnosis of various male reproductive tract infections, including epididymitis, prostatitis, and testicular cancer. This test can also identify any abnormalities in the size, shape, and structure of the male reproductive organs, such as cysts or tumors [27].

X-ray

X-ray is a type of imaging test that uses radiation to produce images of the internal organs and tissues. X-rays are commonly used to diagnose conditions such as testicular torsion, a condition where the testicle twists and cuts off blood supply. X-rays are a non-invasive test that is performed externally by passing radiation through the body and capturing images on film or a digital sensor. X-rays can help in the diagnosis of various male reproductive tract infections, including testicular torsion and tumors [28].

Scrotal Doppler Ultrasound

Scrotal Doppler ultrasound is a type of ultrasonography that uses sound waves to evaluate the blood flow in the scrotum. This test is commonly used to diagnose conditions such as testicular torsion and epididymitis. Scrotal Doppler ultrasound can help in the diagnosis of various male reproductive tract infections, including epididymitis, testicular torsion, and varicocele. This test can also identify any abnormalities in the blood flow to the male reproductive organs [29].

Thus, imaging tests play an essential role in the diagnosis of male reproductive tract infections. These tests can provide valuable information regarding the condition of the male reproductive system and help in the identification of any potential abnormalities or infections.

TREATMENT OF MALE REPRODUCTIVE TRACT INFECTION

In the clinical management of male reproductive tract infections (MRTIs), judicious employment of antimicrobial agents is quintessential. MRTIs encompass a spectrum of conditions, such as prostatitis, epididymitis, and urethritis, and may be caused by a diversity of pathogens, including bacteria, viruses, and fungi. The pharmacological agents primarily used for the treatment include antibiotics, antiviral, and antifungal drugs Fig. (**11**).

Antibiotics, Antiviral and Antifungal Drugs

Antibiotics

Antibiotics are integral to the therapeutic intervention of bacterial infections affecting the male genital tract. The selection of an antibiotic is contingent upon the ascertainment of the pathogenic microorganism and its antimicrobial susceptibility pattern. Fluoroquinolones, including agents like ciprofloxacin and levofloxacin, are often the drugs of choice due to their extensive spectrum of antibacterial activity and superior penetration into tissues, which renders them highly effective in managing ailments such as chronic bacterial prostatitis. In contrast, for the treatment of acute bacterial prostatitis and epididymitis, the utilization of cephalosporins (for instance, ceftriaxone) and doxycycline is considered appropriate. It is critical to customize the antibiotic regimen in accordance with culture findings to thwart the development of antimicrobial resistance [30].

Antiviral Drugs

Viruses, including herpes simplex virus (HSV) and human papillomavirus (HPV), possess the capability to impact the male genital tract. To mitigate the effects of HSV infections, antiviral pharmaceuticals like acyclovir and valacyclovir are utilized. These compounds are categorized as nucleoside analogs, and they function by impeding the viral DNA polymerase enzyme, thereby constraining the replication of the viral genetic material. In cases of HPV infections, which are associated with the manifestation of anogenital warts, topical therapeutic agents such as imiquimod or podophyllin may be administered. Moreover, as a preventive measure, immunization against HPV is advocated to diminish the likelihood of contracting the infection [31].

Antifungal Drugs

Mycotic infections, albeit relatively infrequent, have the potential to impinge upon the male genital tract. Species of the genus Candida are principally implicated in these infections and can precipitate balanitis. The primary intervention usually encompasses the application of topical antifungal medications, including clotrimazole or miconazole. In instances where the infection is intransigent or of a severe nature, it may become imperative to administer systemic antifungal agents like fluconazole [32, 33].

Consequently, addressing infections in the male reproductive tract demands an integrative strategy, employing antibacterial, antiviral, and antifungal medications contingent upon the causative organism. The selection of therapeutic agents is informed by the patient's medical history, clinical manifestations, and diagnostic evaluations. Adherence to the tenets of antimicrobial stewardship is imperative to curtail the emergence of drug-resistant microorganisms and to guarantee the effectiveness of treatment protocols for male reproductive tract infections.

Pain Relief Medication

Within the context of an all-encompassing therapeutic regimen, the dispensation of pain-alleviating pharmaceuticals is paramount in controlling discomfort and pain associated with Male Reproductive Tract Infections (MRTIs). Commonly used as primary pain management drugs for MRTIs are Nonsteroidal Anti-Inflammatory Drugs (NSAIDs) [34]. NSAIDs, including naproxen and ibuprofen, function through the inhibition of cyclooxygenase enzymes (COX-1 and COX-2), which subsequently leads to a reduction in the production of prostaglandins. These are biochemical intermediaries implicated in pain sensation and inflammation initiation. By limiting the synthesis of prostaglandins, NSAIDs can effectively alleviate inflammation and pain within the male reproductive system. However, it is of great importance to monitor the dose as NSAIDs can precipitate adverse effects related to the gastrointestinal, renal, and cardiovascular systems. Another commonly utilized analgesic is acetaminophen, also known as paracetamol, which exhibits a distinct mode of action. Despite the exact mechanism of action not being entirely understood, it is hypothesized that acetaminophen operates centrally in the brain to suppress prostaglandin synthesis without producing significant anti-inflammatory effects. As a consequence, acetaminophen is particularly useful for the management of pain, and its relatively benign side effect profile makes it a potential substitute for patients with NSAID intolerance [34]. For instances of extreme pain, medical practitioners might resort to opioid analgesics, such as morphine or codeine. Opioids act on opioid receptors in the central nervous system to modulate the perception of pain. Due to their potential for dependence and serious side effects like respiratory depression, opioids are typically reserved for situations where non-opioid analgesics are inadequate for pain control.

In cases where MRTIs are a result of bacterial infections, simultaneous administration of suitable antibiotics is essential to address the root cause. This strategy aids in the resolution of the infection, potentially reducing inflammation and pain in the reproductive tract. In addition, patients might be recommended to use supplementary therapies such as cold packs, sitz baths, and scrotal elevation to alleviate scrotal or perineal pain linked with MRTIs. Thus, the management of pain in the context of male reproductive tract infections is complex, necessitating the careful selection of analgesic medications, from NSAIDs and acetaminophen to opioids for more severe cases. This is complemented by addressing the root infection with antibiotics and employing additional pain relief strategies, which are crucial for a comprehensive approach to patient care.

Anti-inflammatory Medication

Among the diversity of therapeutic approaches, the utilization of anti-inflammatory pharmaceuticals is an essential element in the management of MRTIs. Anti-inflammatory pharmaceuticals, encompassing nonsteroidal anti-inflammatory drugs (NSAIDs) and corticosteroids, can play a crucial role in attenuating the inflammatory reaction commonly precipitated during MRTIs. They are designed to act on inflammatory pathways, thus dampening the secretion of inflammatory mediators such as prostaglandins and leukotrienes, which are associated with pain and fluid accumulation in MRTIs [30, 34].

Nonsteroidal anti-inflammatory drugs like ibuprofen and naproxen operate by hindering the activity of cyclooxygenase enzymes (COX-1 and COX-2), consequently suppressing the synthesis of prostaglandins. The suppression of prostaglandins aids in the reduction of pain, edema, and fever – a symptom cluster frequently concomitant with MRTIs. However, the application of NSAIDs necessitates prudence, taking into account potential side effects encompassing gastrointestinal distress, renal dysfunction, and the aggravation of hypertension [34].

Conversely, corticosteroids such as prednisone are powerful anti-inflammatory substances that influence the transcription of genes that are implicated in inflammatory processes. They suppress the expression of a variety of cytokines and adhesion molecules, thus decreasing leukocyte migration and curtailing tissue inflammation. Corticosteroids might be utilized in cases of intense inflammation or where NSAIDs are not advisable [14]. However, it is critical to recognize that corticosteroid therapy comes with risks, and extended application can result in immunosuppression, elevated blood sugar levels, osteoporosis, and other systemic adverse effects. Additionally, the simultaneous application of antibiotics is critical when a bacterial infection is identified as the cause of the MRTI. For example, bacterial prostatitis requires the combined administration of antibiotics and anti-inflammatory drugs to effectively neutralize the infection and subdue the inflammatory response. The choice of antibiotics should hinge on the suspected or verified microbial agent and its susceptibility to antimicrobial agents. Patients receiving treatment for MRTIs should be rigorously supervised to assess clinical responses and potential medication-induced adverse effects. In instances where the condition is unresponsive to pharmacological treatment, or structural anomalies are a contributing factor, surgical intervention may be necessary. Thus, anti-inflammatory pharmaceuticals, encompassing NSAIDs and corticosteroids, are fundamental in the handling of MRTIs. Their role is to curtail inflammation, relieve pain, and forestall complications. Nevertheless, medical practitioners must judiciously balance the advantages with the potential adverse consequences and, when required, incorporate additional therapeutic approaches such as antibiotics for all-encompassing management. Patient instruction and vigilant supervision are crucial constituents of effective treatment protocols [14, 34].

Surgery

Surgical intervention is typically reserved for severe or complicated cases of male reproductive tract infections that do not respond to conservative measures or require direct intervention to address underlying anatomical abnormalities. While many of these infections can be effectively managed without surgery, there are specific situations where surgical interventions may be necessary.

Epididymo-orchitis, which involves inflammation of the epididymis and testicles, is one such condition that may require surgical intervention. When there is the formation of an abscess or a significant accumulation of pus, surgical drainage becomes necessary to remove the infected material and prevent further complications. This procedure, known as scrotal abscess drainage, involves making an incision in the scrotum to access the abscess and evacuate its contents. It is typically performed under anesthesia and followed by a course of antibiotics to eradicate the infection [35, 36].

Chronic prostatitis, particularly when abscesses form or prostate stones are present, may also require surgical intervention. Prostate abscesses often necessitate drainage through procedures such as transrectal ultrasound-guided needle aspiration or transurethral resection of the prostate (TURP). TURP involves removing part of the prostate gland to alleviate obstruction and improve urinary flow. It is considered when chronic prostatitis does not respond to medical management [37].

In rare cases, surgical treatment may be necessary for sexually transmitted infections (STIs) that have caused complications in the male reproductive tract. Advanced syphilis or chancroid may require surgical excision of ulcers or lymph nodes to control the infection. Similarly, severe cases of recurrent genital herpes that do not respond to antiviral medications may require surgical removal of the affected tissue [38, 39].

It is important to emphasize that surgical interventions for male reproductive tract infections are only used for specific indications and are not the primary approach in most cases. Non-surgical treatments, such as antimicrobial therapy, supportive care, and lifestyle modifications, are usually effective in managing these infections. However, surgical intervention can be crucial when conservative measures fail or complications arise. Like any surgical procedure, there are potential risks and complications associated with surgical treatment for male reproductive tract infections, including infection, bleeding, anesthesia-related issues, and damage to surrounding structures [22]. Therefore, the decision to undergo surgery should be made after careful consideration of the individual patient's condition, overall health, and the expertise of the surgical team.

RELATIONSHIP BETWEEN MALE REPRODUCTIVE TRACT INFECTIONS AND INFERTILITY

Effect of Infections on Sperm Production

The correlation between infections in the male reproductive tract and infertility has garnered substantial scientific attention. Infections within the male reproductive system can have adverse consequences on various aspects of reproductive function, particularly sperm production. Infections can disrupt spermatogenesis at multiple levels. One of the primary effects of infections on sperm production is the impairment of testicular function. Inflammatory responses instigated by infections can induce testicular damage, characterized by the infiltration of immune cells and the release of pro-inflammatory molecules [2, 39]. These inflammatory changes can disturb the intricate environment within the testes, which is essential for the generation and maturation of sperm cells. Moreover, infections can directly impact the seminiferous tubules, which are the structures within the testes where spermatogenesis transpires. The presence of pathogens can lead to structural damage, impeding the proper operation of these tubules. Infections can also disrupt the delicate balance of hormones and signaling molecules involved in regulating spermatogenesis, thereby further compromising sperm production [4, 40].

Certain specific infections have been implicated in causing significant harm to sperm production. Sexually transmitted infections (STIs) such as *Chlamydia trachomatis* and *Neisseria gonorrhoeae* can ascend through the male reproductive tract and provoke epididymitis, inflammation of the epididymis [23]. The epididymis plays a crucial role in the maturation and storage of sperm, and inflammation in this region can disrupt the normal maturation process and impair sperm function. In addition to direct effects on sperm production, infections can also influence sperm quality. Inflammatory processes triggered by infections can induce oxidative stress within the testes. Oxidative stress arises when there is an imbalance between the production of reactive oxygen species (ROS) and the ability of the body to neutralize them. Elevated levels of ROS can induce damage to sperm DNA, proteins, and lipids, resulting in diminished sperm motility and viability [41].

It is important to note that not all male reproductive tract infections lead to infertility. The severity and duration of the infection, as well as individual variations in susceptibility, can influence the extent of damage to sperm production [4]. Prompt and appropriate treatment of infections is crucial in order to minimize the potential negative impact on fertility. Thus, infections in the male reproductive tract can have a significant impact on sperm production and contribute to infertility. These infections can impair testicular function, disrupt the seminiferous tubules, and induce oxidative stress, ultimately affecting sperm quality and viability. Comprehending the effects of infections on male fertility can aid in the development of effective preventive measures and treatment strategies to mitigate the risk of infertility associated with reproductive tract infections [40].

Effect of Infections on Semen Quality

Extensive research has been conducted to examine the association between infections in the male reproductive tract and infertility, revealing noteworthy repercussions on the quality of spermatozoa. Infections have the potential to adversely affect various aspects of sperm parameters, thereby leading to impaired fertility. One of the primary consequences of infections on sperm quality involves the modification of sperm concentration [42]. Infections occurring within the male reproductive tract can incite inflammation and obstruct the ducts, thereby impeding the normal flow of spermatozoa. Consequently, a reduced sperm count, scientifically referred to as oligospermia, may occur. Numerous studies have reported a positive correlation between infections such as epididymitis, orchitis, and sexually transmitted infections (STIs), and a decrease in sperm concentration. Moreover, infections can exert deleterious effects on sperm motility, which pertains to the capacity of sperm cells to swim and navigate effectively toward the egg [43, 44]. The inflammatory processes triggered by infections can disrupt the structure and function of the sperm tail, thereby impairing its ability to propel forward. Consequently, individuals afflicted with infections may experience asthenozoospermia, characterized by reduced sperm motility. Research indicates that pathogens such as *Chlamydia trachomatis* and *Mycoplasma genitalium* can directly impact sperm motility, thereby contributing to infertility.

Sperm morphology, encompassing the shape and structure of spermatozoa, represents another crucial parameter that infections can affect [45]. Infections have the potential to induce oxidative stress and trigger the release of reactive oxygen species (ROS), which can inflict damage on the sperm membrane and DNA. Such oxidative damage can result in abnormal sperm morphology, a condition referred to as teratozoospermia. Studies have demonstrated a positive correlation between infections, particularly those caused by bacteria such as *Escherichia coli*, and an increased prevalence of abnormal sperm morphology [46, 47].

Apart from these direct effects on sperm quality, infections can also influence the composition of seminal fluid [17]. Inflammatory responses incited by infections can induce alterations in the composition of seminal plasma, leading to changes in pH levels, enzyme activity, and immune factors. These alterations can further impact sperm function and viability. It is important to note that the severity of these effects may vary depending on factors such as the specific pathogen involved, the duration and intensity of the infection, and individual factors, including immune response [42]. Nevertheless, it is evident that infections occurring in the male reproductive tract can significantly compromise the quality of spermatozoa, thereby contributing to infertility. Therefore, infections in the male reproductive tract have substantial implications for sperm quality and play a significant role in male infertility. They can affect sperm concentration, motility, morphology, and seminal fluid composition. A comprehensive understanding of the impact of infections on sperm parameters is crucial for the diagnosis and treatment of infertility cases associated with infections in the male reproductive tract. Further research is necessary to explore preventive measures, effective treatments, and strategies to mitigate the adverse effects of infections on male fertility.

Effect of Infections on Sperm Motility

Epididymitis, which refers to the inflammation of the epididymis—a convoluted tubule situated on the posterior aspect of the testes where sperm undergo maturation and storage—is a prevalent infection associated with compromised sperm motility [43]. This condition can arise from sexually transmitted infections like gonorrhea or chlamydia, as well as urinary tract infections. Inflammatory responses elicited by these infections can disrupt the normal microenvironment of the epididymis and hinder sperm motility. Furthermore, the generation of inflammatory mediators may induce oxidative stress, further compromising the functionality and motility of spermatozoa [41]. Another significant infection that negatively affects sperm motility is prostatitis, characterized by the inflammation of the prostate gland. Prostatitis can be caused by bacterial infections, and the ensuing inflammation can have an adverse impact on sperm motility. The prostate gland produces seminal fluid, which provides nourishment and a conducive *milieu* for sperm survival and motility. Inflammation disrupts the composition and quality of seminal fluid, impeding sperm movement and reducing their ability to reach and fertilize the ovum [37, 48].

Sexually transmitted infections (STIs) such as gonorrhea, chlamydia, and mycoplasma infections can also directly impair sperm motility. These infections can induce inflammation and harm the male reproductive tract, including the epididymis, vas deferens, and seminal vesicles, which are all integral to sperm transport and function. Moreover, the presence of infectious agents in semen can exert a direct toxic effect on sperm cells, hindering their motility [23, 35, 36].

It is noteworthy that the impact of infections on sperm motility can vary depending on the severity and duration of the infection, as well as individual factors. In certain instances, the effects on motility may be reversible with appropriate treatment and management of the underlying infection [43, 49]. However, persistent or recurrent infections can lead to long-term damage and irreversible reduction in sperm motility, thereby contributing to infertility. Thus, infections affecting the male reproductive tract can significantly impede sperm motility, a critical factor for successful fertilization. Inflammation, oxidative stress, and damage caused by infections can disrupt the normal functioning of reproductive organs involved in sperm production, maturation, and transport [2]. Accurate diagnosis, treatment, and prevention of these infections are imperative for preserving male fertility and addressing the issue of infertility associated with impaired sperm motility.

Effect of Infections on the Reproductive System

The male reproductive system is vulnerable to various infections that can significantly affect its normal functioning and potentially lead to infertility. Infections can impact different components of the male reproductive tract, including the testes, epididymis, seminal vesicles, prostate, and urethra. These infections can arise from bacteria, viruses, fungi, or parasites, and their effects on fertility vary depending on the specific pathogen and the severity of the infection [1, 2]. Epididymitis is a common infection that can impair male fertility. It refers to inflammation of the epididymis, often caused by sexually transmitted infections (STIs) such as Chlamydia trachomatis and Neisseria gonorrhoeae. Epididymitis can lead to scarring and blockage of the epididymal ducts, hindering the transport of sperm from the testes to the ejaculatory ducts. As a result, sperm quality, motility, and concentration may be reduced, ultimately affecting fertility [35, 36]. Prostatitis, an inflammation of the prostate gland, is another significant infection associated with male infertility. Bacterial infections can cause prostatitis, leading to the accumulation of inflammatory cells and impairing prostate function. The presence of bacteria in the semen can negatively impact sperm quality and function. Chronic prostatitis is also linked to the presence of leukocytes in semen, which can contribute to oxidative stress and damage sperm DNA, further compromising fertility [50, 51].

Sexually transmitted infections such as gonorrhea and syphilis can directly affect the testes, leading to orchitis. Orchitis involves testicular inflammation and can result in testicular damage and impaired sperm production [23]. Similarly, infections like mumps, contracted during adolescence or adulthood, can cause orchitis and potentially result in permanent testicular damage. Urinary tract infections (UTIs) can ascend to the male reproductive tract and cause urethritis, affecting the urethra. Urethritis can lead to discomfort and pain during ejaculation, and the inflammatory response can impact sperm quality and function. Infections in the male reproductive tract can disrupt the hormonal environment necessary for normal sperm production. Inflammatory processes triggered by infections can generate reactive oxygen species, impairing sperm function and causing oxidative stress. Additionally, the immune response to infections can produce antibodies that target sperm, further compromising fertility [39].

It is crucial to emphasize that the severity and duration of the infection, as well as timely and appropriate treatment, play a critical role in the potential impact on fertility. Timely diagnosis and management of reproductive tract infections are essential to minimize the risk of infertility [10]. Preventive measures, including safe sexual practices and proper hygiene, are also vital in reducing the incidence of infections and their associated complications on male reproductive health.

PREVENTION OF MALE REPRODUCTIVE TRACT INFECTIONS

The prioritization of male reproductive tract infection prevention holds paramount significance in safeguarding the holistic welfare and reproductive health of individuals. Through the implementation of diverse strategies encompassing prudent sexual conduct, meticulous hygiene protocols, periodic medical examinations, and appropriate immunization, a notable decline in the occurrence of male reproductive tract infections can be attained. This segment will expound upon each of these aspects comprehensively.

Safe Sex Practices

The adoption of safe sexual practices holds paramount importance in the prevention of sexually transmitted infections (STIs) that can impact the male reproductive system. The consistent and accurate utilization of condoms during sexual intercourse serves as a physical barrier, impeding the exchange of bodily fluids harboring pathogenic microorganisms. Furthermore, condoms play a pivotal role in diminishing the likelihood of contracting and transmitting STIs, including gonorrhea, chlamydia, syphilis, and HIV. It is crucial to acknowledge that while condoms offer substantial protection, they do not confer absolute immunity against all types of STIs. Hence, engaging in monogamous relationships, where both partners have undergone STI testing and have been confirmed to be uninfected, further augments the implementation of safe sexual practices [52].

Hygiene Practices

Ensuring adequate hygiene practices is imperative for the prevention of male reproductive tract infections. Consistently cleansing the genital region utilizing gentle soap and warm water facilitates the elimination of dirt, perspiration, and bacteria, thereby diminishing the likelihood of infection. It is crucial to recognize that excessive utilization of potent soaps or abrasive cleansing agents may disrupt the inherent microbial equilibrium in the genital area, potentially resulting in infections. Additionally, it is recommended to don fresh, breathable undergarments composed of natural textiles to enhance optimal airflow and diminish moisture accumulation, thereby mitigating the favorable conditions conducive to bacterial or fungal proliferation [53].

Regular Check-ups

Regular consultations with healthcare professionals play a pivotal role in the detection and prevention of infections affecting the male reproductive tract. Periodic assessments enable healthcare providers to evaluate the holistic well-being of the reproductive system, identify incipient indicators or manifestations of infections, and administer suitable interventions [54]. Moreover, it is advisable to undergo routine screening for sexually transmitted infections (STIs), particularly for individuals who engage in sexual activities with multiple partners or participate in behaviors that heighten their susceptibility to such infections. Timely identification and expeditious treatment of infections significantly mitigate the likelihood of complications and further transmission.

Immunizations

Immunizations play a pivotal role in the prevention of specific infections that can impact the male reproductive tract. Vaccines, such as the human papillomavirus (HPV) vaccine, provide protection against HPV, a prevalent viral infection that can result in the development of genital warts and various types of cancers, including penile, anal, and oropharyngeal cancers. It is recommended that both males and females receive HPV vaccination prior to engaging in sexual activity, as the greatest benefits are achieved when the vaccine is administered before exposure to the virus. By effectively preventing HPV infections, the risk of associated complications affecting the reproductive tract can be significantly mitigated [55, 56].

Therefore, the prevention of infections in the male reproductive tract encompasses a range of strategies that promote safe sexual practices, maintain appropriate hygiene, encourage regular medical examinations, and advocate for immunizations. The implementation of these preventive measures not only decreases the likelihood of acquiring and transmitting infections but also contributes to the overall reproductive health and well-being of individuals. It is imperative for individuals to proactively adopt these practices and seek guidance from healthcare professionals to ensure optimal reproductive health.

CONCLUSION

This chapter has emphasized the importance of male reproductive tract infections (RTIs) in relation to male infertility, highlighting their significant impact on reproductive health. A comprehensive understanding of the diagnosis and treatment of these infections is crucial for effectively managing and preventing infertility in males.

The significance of male reproductive tract infections in male infertility has been underscored in this study. The intricate anatomical and physiological characteristics of the male reproductive system render it vulnerable to a range of infections, including sexually transmitted infections (STIs) and non-sexually transmitted infections. These infections can have detrimental effects on sperm production, motility, and function, ultimately impairing fertility. Additionally, RTIs have been associated with testicular inflammation, oxidative stress, and DNA damage in sperm, further exacerbating infertility. Therefore, it is imperative to recognize the importance of male reproductive tract infections in addressing the complex issue of male infertility.

Early identification and prompt treatment of male reproductive tract infections are essential for mitigating their adverse effects on male fertility. Timely detection of infections through comprehensive diagnostic approaches, such as microbiological culture, molecular testing, and semen analysis, enables healthcare professionals to initiate appropriate treatment strategies promptly. Effective treatment options include tailored antimicrobial therapies targeting the specific causative pathogen, along with supportive measures to alleviate inflammation and enhance reproductive parameters. By addressing infections at an early stage, the potential for irreversible damage to the male reproductive system can be minimized, thereby increasing the likelihood of successful conception.

Prevention strategies play a crucial role in reducing the incidence and burden of male reproductive tract infections, consequently mitigating their negative impact on male fertility. Comprehensive prevention efforts should emphasize safe sexual practices, such as consistent condom usage and regular screenings for STIs. Public health initiatives should also focus on increasing awareness about the risks associated with untreated infections, promoting responsible sexual behavior, and advocating for STI vaccination where available. Moreover, healthcare providers should actively engage in counseling patients regarding risk factors, hygiene practices, and the importance of seeking timely medical care for suspected infections.

Effectively managing male reproductive tract infections is intricately linked to addressing male infertility. Recognizing the significance of these infections, ensuring early diagnosis and appropriate treatment, and implementing effective prevention strategies are vital steps in safeguarding male reproductive health and promoting successful reproductive outcomes. By adopting a comprehensive approach that encompasses clinical, research, and public health efforts, we can work towards reducing the burden of male infertility caused by reproductive tract infections, ultimately improving the quality of life for individuals and couples affected by this challenging condition.

REFERENCES

[1]   Narvekar S. Microbiology of Semen and Male Genital Tract Infections. 2013.

[2]   Sengupta P, Dutta S, Alahmar AT. Reproductive tract infection, inflammation and male infertility. Chem Biol Lett 2020; 7: 75-84.

[3]   Agarwal A, Mulgund A, Hamada A, Chyatte MR. A unique view on male infertility around the globe. Reprod Biol Endocrinol 2015; 13(1): 37.
[http://dx.doi.org/10.1186/s12958-015-0032-1] [PMID: 25928197]

[4]   Dutta S, Sengupta P, Chhikara BS. Reproductive inflammatory mediators and male infertility. Chem Biol Lett 2020; 7: 73-4.

[5]   Pellati D, Mylonakis I, Bertoloni G, *et al.* Genital tract infections and infertility. Eur J Obstet Gynecol Reprod Biol 2008; 140(1): 3-11.
[http://dx.doi.org/10.1016/j.ejogrb.2008.03.009] [PMID: 18456385]

[6]   Workowski KA, Bachmann LH, Chan PA, Johnston CM, Muzny CA, Park I, *et al.* Sexually Transmitted Infections Treatment Guidelines, 2021. MMWR Recommendations and reports : Morbidity and mortality weekly report Recommendations and reports. 2021; 70: 1-187.

[7]   Richardson MD, Warnock DW. Fungal infection: diagnosis and management. John Wiley & Sons 2012.
[http://dx.doi.org/10.1002/9781118321492]

[8]   Rivero MJ, Kulkarni N, Thirumavalavan N, Ramasamy R. Evaluation and management of male genital tract infections in the setting of male infertility: an updated review. Curr Opin Urol 2023; 33(3): 180-6.
[http://dx.doi.org/10.1097/MOU.0000000000001081] [PMID: 36861760]

[9]   Tonolini M, Ippolito S. Cross-sectional imaging of complicated urinary infections affecting the lower

tract and male genital organs. Insights Imaging 2016; 7(5): 689-711.
[http://dx.doi.org/10.1007/s13244-016-0503-8] [PMID: 27271509]

[10]   Purvis K, Christiansen E. Infection in the male reproductive tract. Impact, diagnosis and treatment in relation to male infertility. Int J Androl 1993; 16(1): 1-13.
[http://dx.doi.org/10.1111/j.1365-2605.1993.tb01146.x] [PMID: 8468091]

[11]   Assi R, Hashim PW, Reddy VB, Einarsdottir H, Longo WE. Sexually transmitted infections of the anus and rectum. World J Gastroenterol 2014; 20(41): 15262-8.
[http://dx.doi.org/10.3748/wjg.v20.i41.15262] [PMID: 25386074]

[12]   Dohle GR. Inflammatory-associated obstructions of the male reproductive tract. Andrologia 2003; 35(5): 321-4.
[http://dx.doi.org/10.1111/j.1439-0272.2003.tb00866.x] [PMID: 14535864]

[13]   Agarwal A, Finelli R, Durairajanayagam D, *et al.* Comprehensive analysis of global research on human varicocele: a scientometric approach. World J Mens Health 2022; 40(4): 636-52.
[http://dx.doi.org/10.5534/wjmh.210202] [PMID: 35118839]

[14]   Haidl G, Haidl F, Allam JP, Schuppe HC. Therapeutic options in male genital tract inflammation. Andrologia 2019; 51(3): e13207.
[http://dx.doi.org/10.1111/and.13207] [PMID: 30474250]

[15]   Leisegang K, Dutta S. Do lifestyle practices impede male fertility? Andrologia 2021; 53(1): e13595.
[http://dx.doi.org/10.1111/and.13595] [PMID: 32330362]

[16]   Naber KG, Bergman B, Bishop MC, *et al.* EAU guidelines for the management of urinary and male genital tract infections. Eur Urol 2001; 40(5): 576-88.
[http://dx.doi.org/10.1159/000049840] [PMID: 11752870]

[17]   Tan CW, Chlebicki MP. Urinary tract infections in adults. Singapore Med J 2016; 57(9): 485-90.
[http://dx.doi.org/10.11622/smedj.2016153] [PMID: 27662890]

[18]   Bourne H, Archer J. Sperm preparation techniques Textbook of assisted reproductive techniques. CRC Press 2017; pp. 92-106.

[19]   Beydola T, Sharma RK, Lee W, Agarwal A, Rizk B, Aziz N, *et al.* Sperm preparation and selection techniques Male Infertility Practice New Delhi. Jaypee Brothers Medical Publishers 2013; pp. 244-51.

[20]   Organization WH. WHO laboratory manual for the examination and processing of human semen. World Health Organization 2021.

[21]   Harrison PE, Barratt CLR, Robinson AJ, Kessopoulou E, Cooke ID. Detection of white blood cell populations in the ejaculates of fertile men. J Reprod Immunol 1991; 19(1): 95-8.
[http://dx.doi.org/10.1016/0165-0378(91)90009-F] [PMID: 2007999]

[22]   Traisman ES. Clinical management of urinary tract infections. Pediatr Ann 2016; 45(4): e108-11.
[http://dx.doi.org/10.3928/00904481-20160316-01] [PMID: 27064464]

[23]   Ochsendorf FR. Sexually transmitted infections: impact on male fertility. Andrologia 2008; 40(2): 72-5.
[http://dx.doi.org/10.1111/j.1439-0272.2007.00825.x] [PMID: 18336453]

[24]   Wallach EE, Wolff H. The biologic significance of white blood cells in semen. Fertil Steril 1995; 63(6): 1143-57.
[http://dx.doi.org/10.1016/S0015-0282(16)57588-8] [PMID: 7750580]

[25]   Steinkeler JA, Sun MR, Eds. Imaging of infections of the urinary and male reproductive tracts Seminars in Roentgenology. Elsevier 2017.

[26]   Lotti F, Maggi M. Ultrasound of the male genital tract in relation to male reproductive health. Hum Reprod Update 2015; 21(1): 56-83.
[http://dx.doi.org/10.1093/humupd/dmu042] [PMID: 25038770]

[27]   El-Ghar MA, Farg H, Sharaf DE, El-Diasty T. CT and MRI in Urinary Tract Infections: A Spectrum of Different Imaging Findings. Medicina (Kaunas) 2021; 57(1): 32.
[http://dx.doi.org/10.3390/medicina57010032]

[28]   Abdelmalak JB, Vasavada SP, Rackley RR. Urinary tract infections in adults Essential Urology: A Guide to Clinical Practice. Springer 2004; pp. 183-9.
[http://dx.doi.org/10.1007/978-1-59259-737-6_10]

[29]   Khatri ZA, Sohail S. Gray scale and doppler ultra-sound in the diagnosis of painless scrotal masses. Pak J Med Sci 2010; 26: 178-82.

[30]   Izuka E, Menuba I, Sengupta P, Dutta S, Nwagha U. Antioxidants, anti-inflammatory drugs and antibiotics in the treatment of reproductive tract infections and their association with male infertility. Chem Biol Lett 2020.

[31]   Else LJ, Taylor S, Back DJ, Khoo SH. Pharmacokinetics of antiretroviral drugs in anatomical sanctuary sites: the male and female genital tract. Antivir Ther 2011; 16(8): 1149-67.
[http://dx.doi.org/10.3851/IMP1919] [PMID: 22155899]

[32]   Rapp RP. Changing strategies for the management of invasive fungal infections. Pharmacotherapy 2004; 24(2P2): 4S-28S.
[http://dx.doi.org/10.1592/phco.24.3.4S.33151] [PMID: 14992487]

[33]   Gupta AK, Sauder DN, Shear NH. Antifungal agents: An overview. Part II. J Am Acad Dermatol 1994; 30(6): 911-33.
[http://dx.doi.org/10.1016/S0190-9622(94)70112-1] [PMID: 7619094]

[34]   Panchal NK, Prince Sabina E. Non-steroidal anti-inflammatory drugs (NSAIDs): A current insight into its molecular mechanism eliciting organ toxicities. Food Chem Toxicol 2023; 172: 113598.
[http://dx.doi.org/10.1016/j.fct.2022.113598] [PMID: 36608735]

[35]   Krieger JN. Epididymitis, orchitis, and related conditions. Sex Transmit Dis 1984; pp. 173-81.

[36]   Banyra O, Shulyak A. URINARY TRACT INFECTION Acute epididymo-orchitis: staging and treatment. Cent European J Urol 2012; 65(3): 139-43.
[http://dx.doi.org/10.5173/ceju.2012.03.art8] [PMID: 24578950]

[37]   Schoeb DS, Schlager D, Boeker M, *et al.* Surgical therapy of prostatitis: a systematic review. World J Urol 2017; 35(11): 1659-68.
[http://dx.doi.org/10.1007/s00345-017-2054-0] [PMID: 28612108]

[38]   Radhakrishna K Problematic ulcerative lesions in sexually transmitted diseases: surgical management. Sex Transmit Dis 1986; pp. 127-33.

[39]   Schuppe HC, Pilatz A, Hossain H, Diemer T, Wagenlehner F, Weidner W. Urogenital infection as a risk factor for male infertility. Dtsch Arztebl Int 2017; 114(19): 339-46.
[http://dx.doi.org/10.3238/arztebl.2017.0339] [PMID: 28597829]

[40]   Dutta S, Sengupta P, Slama P, Roychoudhury S. Oxidative stress, testicular inflammatory pathways, and male reproduction. Int J Mol Sci 2021; 22(18): 10043.
[http://dx.doi.org/10.3390/ijms221810043] [PMID: 34576205]

[41]   Dutta S, Sengupta P, Chakravarthi S. Oxidant-Sensitive Inflammatory Pathways and Male Reproductive Functions Oxidative Stress and Toxicity in Reproductive Biology and Medicine: A Comprehensive Update on Male Infertility-Volume One. Springer 2022; pp. 165-80.
[http://dx.doi.org/10.1007/978-3-030-89340-8_8]

[42]   Irez T, Bicer S, Sahin S, Dutta S, Sengupta P. Cytokines and adipokines in the regulation of spermatogenesis and semen quality. Chem Biol Lett 2020; 7: 131-9.

[43]   Diemer T, Huwe P, Ludwig M, Hauck EW, Weidner W. Urogenital infection and sperm motility. Andrologia 2003; 35(5): 283-7.
[http://dx.doi.org/10.1111/j.1439-0272.2003.tb00858.x] [PMID: 14535856]

[44] Köhn FM, Erdmann I, Oeda T, Mulla KFE, Schiefer HG, Schill WB. Influence of urogenital infections on sperm functions. Andrologia 1998; 30(S1) (Suppl. 1): 73-80.
[http://dx.doi.org/10.1111/j.1439-0272.1998.tb02829.x] [PMID: 9629446]

[45] Menkveld R, Kruger TF. Sperm morphology and male urogenital infections. Andrologia 1998; 30(S1) (Suppl. 1): 49-53.
[http://dx.doi.org/10.1111/j.1439-0272.1998.tb02826.x] [PMID: 9629443]

[46] Kaur K, Prabha V. Sperm impairment by sperm agglutinating factor isolated from Escherichia coli: Receptor specific interactions. BioMed Res Int. 2013; 2013.

[47] Bussalleu E, Yeste M, Sepúlveda L, Torner E, Pinart E, Bonet S. Effects of different concentrations of enterotoxigenic and verotoxigenic E. coli on boar sperm quality. Anim Reprod Sci 2011; 127(3-4): 176-82.
[http://dx.doi.org/10.1016/j.anireprosci.2011.07.018] [PMID: 21907505]

[48] Meinhardt A, Hedger MP. Immunological, paracrine and endocrine aspects of testicular immune privilege. Mol Cell Endocrinol 2011; 335(1): 60-8.
[http://dx.doi.org/10.1016/j.mce.2010.03.022] [PMID: 20363290]

[49] Gaffney EA, Gadêlha H, Smith DJ, Blake JR, Kirkman-Brown JC. Mammalian sperm motility: observation and theory. Annu Rev Fluid Mech 2011; 43(1): 501-28.
[http://dx.doi.org/10.1146/annurev-fluid-121108-145442]

[50] Osadchuk LV, Erkovich AA, Tataru DA, Markova EV, Svetlakov AV. [Level of DNA fragmentation in human sperm cells in varicocele and prostatitis]. Urologiia 2014; (3): 37-43.
[PMID: 25211925]

[51] Casey HW, Irving GW. Bacterial, Mycoplasmal, Mycotic, and Immune-Mediated Diseases of the Urogenital System. In: Foster HL, Small JD, Fox JG, Eds. Diseases. Academic Press 1982; pp. 43-53.
[http://dx.doi.org/10.1016/B978-0-12-262502-2.50010-9]

[52] Kippax S. Safe Sex: It's not as Simple as ABC Routledge handbook of sexuality, health and rights. Routledge 2010; pp. 184-92.

[53] Hillier MD. Using effective hand hygiene practice to prevent and control infection. Nurs Stand 2020; 35(5): 45-50.
[http://dx.doi.org/10.7748/ns.2020.e11552] [PMID: 32337862]

[54] Dayan L, Ooi C. The sexually transmitted infection'check up. Austr Fam Phys 2003; p. 32.

[55] Stanberry LR, Cunningham AL, Mindel A, *et al.* Prospects for control of herpes simplex virus disease through immunization. Clin Infect Dis 2000; 30(3): 549-66.
[http://dx.doi.org/10.1086/313687] [PMID: 10722443]

[56] St Laurent J, Luckett R, Feldman S. HPV vaccination and the effects on rates of HPV-related cancers. Curr Probl Cancer 2018; 42(5): 493-506.
[http://dx.doi.org/10.1016/j.currproblcancer.2018.06.004] [PMID: 30041818]

SUBJECT INDEX

A

Abnormal sperm 26, 69
  production 26, 69
  shape 26
Abnormalities 10, 11, 19, 26, 34, 45, 69, 87,
    88, 91, 168, 179, 185, 186
  chromosomal 19, 26, 69, 87, 88
  congenital 45
  reproductive 10, 11
Acid, amino 93
Activation 36, 50, 54
  inhibiting T-cell 54
  lymphocyte 50
  of apoptotic pathways 36
Activin 53, 54
Activities 52, 187, 193
  antibacterial 187
  enzyme 193
  inflammatory 52
Acute 100, 101, 123, 124, 165, 187
  bacterial prostatitis 100, 101, 123, 124, 187
  inflammations 165
Air pollution 90
Anabolic steroids 14
Androgen(s) 11, 29, 31, 32, 55
  influence 55
  receptor (AR) 11, 29, 31, 32
  insensitivity syndrome (AIS) 11, 31, 32
Androstenedione 7, 9
Anger, intense 15
Angiogenesis 69
Angiotensin-converting enzyme 145
Anti-inflammatory 46, 51, 85, 93, 113, 177,
    189
  agents 177
  cytokines 46, 51
  medication 113, 189
  properties 93
  therapies 85
Anti-sperm antibody (ASAs) 64, 65, 66, 68,
    74, 75, 76

Antibiotic(s) 93, 94, 101, 102, 105, 109, 112,
    113, 124, 125, 126, 172, 177, 181, 185,
    187, 189, 190
  broad-spectrum 109, 172
  -resistant bacteria 112
  therapy 185
Antibodies 44, 48, 53, 64, 65, 66, 68, 74, 75,
    132, 147, 151, 168, 195
  anti-sperm 64, 68, 75, 147
  male sperm 74
  viral 151
Antifungal 113, 164, 167, 168, 169, 170, 187,
    188
  Agents 164
  drugs 169, 187
  medications 113, 167, 170, 188
  therapy 164, 168, 169
Antigenic properties 48
Antigens, compartmentalize 45
Antileukoprotease 169
Antioxidant 33, 37, 85, 93
  and anti-inflammatory therapies 85
  defenses 33
  -rich foods 93
  supplementation 37, 93
Antipsychotics 14
Antiviral and antifungal drugs 187
Autoimmune 46, 51, 53, 56, 122, 127
  attack 51
  complications 122
  reactions 46, 53, 56, 127

B

Bacterial infections 128, 131
  effects of 131
  transmitted 128
Bacterial lipopolysaccharides 131
Bacterial prostatitis 101, 124, 189
  treatment for acute 101, 124
  treatment for chronic 101, 124
Benign prostatic hyperplasia (BPH) 110

www.ingramcontent.com/pod-product-compliance
Lightning Source LLC
Chambersburg PA
CBHW050840220326
41598CB00006B/412